Silent Killers

From Arsenic to Strychnine

A History of Poison

Stella Berry

If you would like to be informed when future books by this author are released, please sign up to the Reader Group at www.stellaberrybooks.com

Copyright © Stella Berry 2024

All rights reserved. This book or any portion thereof may not be reproduced or used in any manner without the express written permission of the publisher or author except for the use of brief quotations in a book review.

Contents

1. Introduction 5
2. The Ancient Art of Poisoning 7
3. Arsenic: The King of Poisons 10
4. Belladonna: Deadly Nightshade's Dark Secrets 16
5. Atropine: The Deadly Double-Edged Sword 21
6. Curare: Paralysis from the Amazon 24
7. Cyanide: A Swift and Silent Killer 31
8. Digitalis: Nature's Heart-stopping Toxin 43
9. Hemlock: The Poison of Philosophers 53
10. Mercury: The Mad Hatter's Nemesis 64
11. Deadly Delicacies: The Perilous World of Poisonous Mushrooms 73
12. Polonium: The Radiant Assassin 84
13. Ricin: Nature's Lethal Protein 94
14. Strychnine: Convulsions and Crime 101
15. Other Notable Poisons and Their Associated Murders or Assassination Attempts 111

    Thallium: The Silent Assassin 111

    Dimethylmercury: A Silent and Deadly Chemical 113

    Dioxin: A Political Poison 116

    VX Nerve Agent: A Lethal Tool in Covert
    Operations 118

    Hydrogen Cyanide: A Chemical With a
    Dark History 121

    Morphine/Heroin: A Tool for a Serial Killer
    in Medicine 124

    Nicotine: A Toxic Agent Beyond Addiction 127

    Botulinum Toxin: From Cosmetic to
    Chemical Weapon 130

16. The Race Against Time: Fighting Poisons
with Science 133

17. Poison in Pop Culture 141

18. The Modern Age of Poisoning 145

19. Conclusion: The Enduring Enigma of Poisons 149

20. Appendix 152

    Glossary of Terms 152

    Timeline of Key Poisoning Incidents 154

    Recommended Reading and Resources 155

    Online Resources 156

1. Introduction

Throughout history, few things have captured the human imagination quite like poison. It's a symbol of power and vulnerability, of treachery and cunning. The mere whisper of the word conjures images of shadowy figures, clandestine meetings, and vengeful plots. Poisons have long been both weapons of assassins and tools of lovers; they've been the quiet accomplices in political intrigues and the subjects of countless tales of mystery and suspense.

The allure of poison lies not only in its deadly potency but also in its duality. On one hand, poisons represent a dark and sinister world, where a single drop or touch can end a life. On the other, they fascinate us, drawing us into tales of forbidden love, espionage, and power plays. The dichotomy between poison's grim reputation and its captivating history is profound. From Cleopatra's rumored suicide by the bite of an asp to the more modern tales of espionage involving radioactive polonium, the narrative of poison is deeply intertwined with our cultural, political, and social fabric.

Yet, for all its dread and allure, poison is also a testament to the ever-evolving understanding of science and the natural world. Many substances that were once employed covertly in the shadows have now found their place in the spotlight, serving as medicines, research tools, and more. The line between a potent poison and a life-saving drug can be incredibly thin, a theme that resonates throughout history and underscores the complex relationship humanity has with these potent substances.

In "Silent Killers: From Arsenic to Strychnine," we will embark on a journey through time, tracing the histories of some of the world's most infamous poisons. Beginning with the ancient and well-known arsenic, we'll explore the tales, myths, and facts surrounding these deadly substances, delving into their chemical properties, their roles in historic events, and their dual potentials for harm and healing. By the time we reach strychnine, a poison synonymous with mystery novels and detective stories, readers will have gained a nuanced understanding of the multifaceted world of toxins.

Our expedition will not just be about the poisons themselves but also about the people who wielded them, the victims who succumbed to them, and the scientists and doctors who worked tirelessly to understand and combat them. Each chapter will shine a light on a specific poison, unraveling its tales of intrigue, its scientific makeup, and its impact on society.

So, as we prepare to delve into this fascinating and sometimes morbid world, let us remember: in the realm of poison, nothing is ever as simple as it seems. The line between friend and foe, between medicine and toxin, is often blurred. And it's this ambiguity, this dance with danger and discovery, that makes the history of poison a tale worth telling.

2. The Ancient Art of Poisoning

The Dawn of Toxicity

Long before the rise of modern science and forensic toxicology, ancient civilizations recognized the power of natural substances to harm or heal. The earliest uses of poisons were likely stumbled upon by observation, trial, and error. Early humans, observing animals, would have noticed the deadly effects certain plants or creatures had on those that consumed them. These initial encounters with toxic substances paved the way for both cautionary tales and cunning applications.

The practice of poisoning dates back thousands of years. Some ancient tribes employed poisons for hunting, using toxic plant extracts to tip their arrows and ensure a kill. Others recognized the medicinal properties of these substances, using them in small doses to treat ailments or induce altered states of consciousness during religious ceremonies.

The Pharaohs and their Final Drink

The ancient Egyptians had a complex relationship with poisons. While they recognized the therapeutic properties of certain toxins, employing them in their early medical practices, there were also tales of treachery within the royal courts. The infamous Cleopatra was known for her fascination with poisons. Legend has it that she tested various toxins on condemned prisoners to understand their effects. Her own demise, while debated by historians, is often attributed to suicide by the bite of an asp, a symbol of divine royalty in ancient Egypt.

The Greeks and their Deadly Draughts

The ancient Greeks, with their advancements in science and philosophy, were not immune to the allure of poisons. Hemlock, a plant native to Europe and parts of Asia, became infamous in Greek history. It's best remembered for its role in the state-sanctioned execution of the philosopher Socrates, who was made to drink a concoction derived from it. Hemlock's potent neurotoxic properties lead to paralysis and, eventually, death.

Rumors and Royals: Notable Victims of the Silent Killers

History is replete with tales of renowned figures meeting their end at the hands of poisons, though it's essential to approach these accounts with a grain of skepticism. The lack of advanced forensic methods in ancient times means that many of these alleged poisonings remain shrouded in mystery and speculation.

- **Emperor Claudius:** The Roman Emperor is believed to have been poisoned by his wife, Agrippina, who wished to see her son Nero ascend to the throne. The rumored agent of death? A dish of deadly mushrooms.

- **Hannibal Barca:** The Carthaginian general, known for his tactical genius against Rome, is said to have ended his life with poison to avoid capture by his enemies.

- **Alexander the Great:** The sudden and mysterious death of one of history's most celebrated conquerors has led to numerous theories. Some historians speculate that he may have been poisoned, though by whom and for what reason remains a topic of debate.

- **Pope Alexander VI:** A member of the notorious Borgia family, his death has often been linked to the very poison he's rumored to have used on his enemies. The truth, however, remains elusive.

As we journey further into the annals of history, we'll find that poisons have played a role in shaping the fate of empires and the destinies of their rulers. The stories that emerge provide a fascinating glimpse into the minds of those who wielded these silent killers, whether for political power, personal gain, or, sometimes, sheer desperation.

3. Arsenic: The King of Poisons

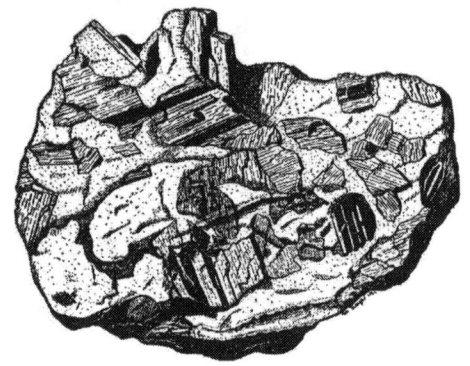

ARSENIC

Historical Sources and Uses

A Natural Killer: Arsenic, a metallic element, has been known since ancient times. Its name, derived from the Greek word "arsenikon", which means 'potent', tells us of its old-world origins. Naturally occurring in the Earth's crust, arsenic can be found in minerals like arsenopyrite, realgar, and orpiment. For ancient civilizations, these minerals, with their vibrant colors, served as pigments in cosmetics and artworks.

Alchemy and Medicine: Beyond its use in art, arsenic, due to its potency, became a staple in the world of alchemy. Alchemists, in their quest to transform base metals into gold, often experimented with arsenic. But it wasn't just the world of mysticism that saw the use of this element. The paradoxical nature of arsenic meant that while it could kill, it was also employed as a medicine. Throughout history, small doses of arsenic were used to treat ailments ranging from ulcers to malaria.

A Silent Tool of Treachery: Given its easy availability and potent effects, arsenic quickly gained notoriety as a favored poison. Its lack of taste and odor made it a discreet weapon, especially in a world devoid of forensic toxicology.

Arsenic in Folk Remedies and Cosmetics

Beyond its malicious use as a silent killer, arsenic found its way into the daily lives of people in ways that might seem astonishing today.

Elixir of Beauty: In the Victorian era, arsenic was hailed as a cosmetic wonder. It was believed that consuming small amounts could improve complexion, giving the skin a paler, more "aristocratic" appearance. Arsenic wafers were sold for this purpose, and though they were consumed in doses deemed "safe," prolonged use led to chronic arsenic poisoning in many.

Arsenic Green: One of the most vivid colors of the 19th century was the emerald shade known as "Scheele's Green" or later "Paris Green." This arsenic-infused pigment adorned wallpapers, dresses, and even candies. Prolonged exposure, especially in damp rooms where the arsenic-laced wallpaper could release toxic fumes, resulted in numerous cases of mysterious illnesses and deaths.

Victorian Arsenic Wafers: Production and Sourcing

- **Mining:** The primary source of arsenic in the Victorian era was from mining. Arsenic is often found as an impurity in metals, such as copper and lead. The Cornwall region of England was a significant producer of arsenic during the 19th century due to its booming tin and copper mining industry. The ore from these mines often contained arsenic, leading to a secondary industry for arsenic extraction and refinement.

- **Production of Wafers:** The exact formulae for arsenic wafers might have varied among manufacturers, but they essentially contained a small, "non-toxic" dose of arsenic combined with filler ingredients to form a wafer or pill. The idea was that these controlled doses would bestow benefits without causing overt poisoning. Over time, however, chronic ingestion could lead to arsenic toxicity.

- **Marketing and Misconceptions:** These wafers were often marketed as health and beauty enhancers. Due to the lack of proper regulation and scientific understanding, the risks of consuming arsenic were vastly underestimated. The paleness induced by arsenic was associated with aristocracy and beauty, making these wafers particularly appealing to women.

Acquisition of Arsenic in More Recent Times

- **Pesticides and Herbicides:** Until the late 20th century, arsenic-based compounds, like lead arsenate, were commonly used as pesticides, especially in orchards. Paris Green, an arsenic-based pigment, was also used as an insecticide. These uses made arsenic relatively accessible.

- **Rat Poison:** Arsenic was a common ingredient in many rat poisons. As such, acquiring arsenic could be as simple as purchasing a readily available poison.

- **Industrial Uses:** Arsenic has had several industrial applications, from the production of glass to electronics. Someone with access to certain industries or knowledge of their processes could potentially acquire arsenic.

- **Regulations and Restrictions:** In modern times, the known dangers of arsenic have led to tighter regulations on its sale and distribution. Many countries have banned or heavily restricted its use in pesticides, and its sale as a raw chemical is often monitored. However, determined individuals could potentially obtain it from less-regulated sources or regions, or from old stocks that pre-date current regulations.

In any era, the potential misuse of arsenic comes down to its dual nature. It has legitimate applications in various industries and historically in medicine, but its lethal potential has often overshadowed these uses. Today's strict regulations reflect a hard-learned understanding of its dangers, but in earlier times, its ready availability led to countless tragedies.

A Slow Killer: The Legacy of Arsenic in Groundwater

One of the most tragic and ongoing arsenic-related crises is the contamination of groundwater, especially in regions of South Asia.

Silent Contamination: In the late 20th century, tube wells were drilled extensively in countries like Bangladesh to provide cleaner drinking water, free from surface water pathogens. However, the drawn groundwater in many areas was found to have naturally high arsenic levels.

A Modern-Day Tragedy: The World Health Organization calls this the "largest mass poisoning of a population in history." Chronic exposure to arsenic in drinking water has resulted in skin lesions, cancers, and various other ailments for millions.

The Science: How Arsenic Affects the Body

A Complex Invader: When ingested, inhaled, or absorbed, arsenic disrupts a multitude of cellular processes. It interferes with over 200 enzymes in the human body, impacting cellular energy production, DNA repair, and various metabolic processes.

Acute and Chronic Poisoning: An immediate and substantial dose of arsenic can lead to acute symptoms like abdominal pain, vomiting, diarrhea, and even death. On the other hand, chronic exposure, even in low amounts, can lead to skin changes, liver disease, diabetes, and an increased risk of cancer.

Detection and Antidotes: By the 19th century, the Marsh test was developed, enabling the detection of arsenic in corpses and providing a means for post-mortem confirmation of arsenical poisoning. In terms of treatment, chelation therapy, using agents like dimercaprol, is employed to bind and eliminate arsenic from the body.

Case Studies: Famous Arsenic Poisonings

- **Napoleon Bonaparte:** One of history's most debated poisonings, traces of arsenic were found in Napoleon's hair after his death. While some believe he was murdered during his exile on St. Helena, others argue that the arsenic came from the environment or was used as a preservative after death.

- **King George III of England:** Known for his bouts of "madness," recent studies suggest that the king might have suffered from chronic arsenic poisoning, with the toxin found in the papers of his personal library.

- **The Bradford Sweets Poisoning:** In 1858, arsenic was mistakenly used as an ingredient in peppermint candies sold in Bradford, England. The error led to the deaths of over 20 people and highlighted the need for stricter food and drug regulations.

4. Belladonna: Deadly Nightshade's Dark Secrets

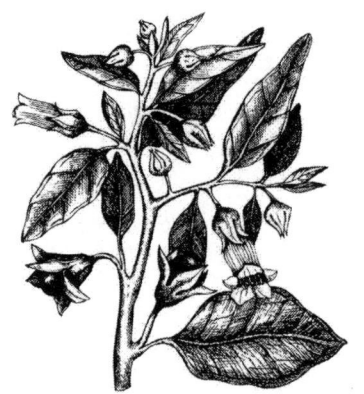

BELLADONNA / DEADLY NIGHTSHADE

Origins and Applications

A Plant of Ancient Roots: Native to Europe, North Africa, and Western Asia, the deadly nightshade, Atropa belladonna, has been recognized and utilized for its potent compounds for millennia. The plant's genus name, "Atropa," is derived from Atropos, one of the three Fates in Greek mythology who was responsible for cutting the thread of life, a nod to the plant's deadly nature.

Beauty and the Belladonna: The name "belladonna" translates to "beautiful lady." During the Renaissance in Italy, women used the juice of the belladonna berries to dilate their pupils, a cosmetic trend of the time, despite the risks involved.

Nature's Deceptive Beauty: Atropa belladonna is a perennial herb with striking purple, bell-shaped flowers and glossy black berries. Its leaves are ovate and the plant stands at a height of around 4 to 5 feet when mature. This deceptive beauty often lures the unsuspecting into considering it harmless.

Geographical Distribution: Belladonna thrives in Europe, North Africa, and Western Asia. Preferring calcareous, chalky soils, it's often found in woodlands and along stream banks.

Extraction of Its Lethal Essence: Traditional extraction of the poison involved drying and grinding the leaves and berries, then using organic solvents to isolate the alkaloids. This method often yields a fine powder or paste which was then used for various purposes. In modern times, more refined chemical techniques are employed, allowing for a purer extraction of compounds like atropine and scopolamine.

Medicine and Myth: Belladonna was employed medicinally for various conditions, from headaches to gastrointestinal disorders. However, the narrow therapeutic window meant that therapeutic use could easily verge on toxic. Moreover, its association with mysticism, as an ingredient in witches' potions and brews, only added to its enigmatic nature.

Legendary Tales and Real Incidents

The Borgia Intrigues: The Borgia family, with their storied history of political machinations during the Renaissance in Italy, is believed to have employed belladonna among other poisons to dispatch rivals and consolidate power.

Julius Caesar and the Conspiracy: There are unverified tales that suggest members of the Roman Senate might have used belladonna as a means to eliminate political adversaries. While most famously associated with the Borgia family, some believe that even individuals close to Julius Caesar might have considered belladonna as an assassination tool.

Agrippina's Ambition: Historical texts hint at Agrippina the Younger, the mother of Nero, having used a mix of belladonna and other poisons to dispatch her rivals and clear her son's path to the Roman throne.

Shakespeare's Potent Brew: While it's speculative, some scholars argue that the potion Juliet consumed in Shakespeare's "Romeo and Juliet" may have contained traces of belladonna, among other ingredients, given the described effects.

Soldiers and Sorcery: In folklore, it was rumored that belladonna was used by ancient warriors to confer fearlessness and strength, though these tales often blur the line between myth and reality.

Mysterious Overdoses: Modern cases often involve individuals accidentally consuming the berries, which can look deceptively inviting, or deliberately ingesting parts of the plant seeking its hallucinogenic properties, only to be overwhelmed by its toxic effects.

The Science Behind the Symptoms

Chemical Constituents: Belladonna's power lies in its tropane alkaloids, primarily atropine, scopolamine, and hyoscyamine. These chemicals are concentrated in the plant's roots, leaves, and seeds.

Mechanism of Action: Belladonna alkaloids are anticholinergics, meaning they block the action of the neurotransmitter acetylcholine. This disrupts the parasympathetic nervous system which is responsible for "rest and digest" activities. Thus, symptoms of poisoning can include a dry mouth, blurred vision, rapid heartbeat, hallucinations, and in severe cases, respiratory failure and death.

From Symptoms to Treatment: Ingestion of belladonna leads to symptoms within just a few hours. Early intervention is critical, and treatments typically involve activated charcoal to prevent further absorption of the poison, as well as supportive therapies like IV fluids and benzodiazepines for seizures.

Conclusion

Belladonna, with its beguiling appearance and potent chemical makeup, has been a subject of both fascination and dread through the ages. From its rumored ties to historical plots of intrigue to its very real and deadly effects, belladonna has carved a niche in the annals of botany, medicine, and history. It serves as a testament to nature's paradoxical ability to nurture and negate life, reminding humanity of the need for respect and caution when treading into the domain of the natural world.

5. Atropine: The Deadly Double-Edged Sword

I have added Atropine to this chapter as it is so closely related to Belladonna, but not the same thing. To clarify:

Atropa Belladonna (Deadly Nightshade):

- **Plant Description:** Belladonna is a perennial herbaceous plant. It has purple, bell-shaped flowers and shiny black berries.

- **Toxins Present:** The plant contains several tropane alkaloids, with the most notable being atropine, scopolamine (hyoscine), and hyoscyamine.

Atropine:

- **Chemical Description:** Atropine is a specific tropane alkaloid compound.

- **Source:** It's one of the primary active components extracted from the belladonna plant, among other plants.

- **Uses:** Atropine has a wide range of medical applications, including use as an antidote for certain types of poisonings (like organophosphate pesticide poisoning), to increase heart rate in cases of bradycardia, and to reduce salivary and bronchial secretions during surgery.

In essence, belladonna is the plant that contains various compounds, including atropine, while atropine itself is a specific chemical compound extracted from the plant.

Atropine's Dual Role as Poison and Antidote

A Fine Line: Atropine, in large doses, can be fatal. It affects various bodily functions, leading to symptoms like dry mouth, blurred vision, hallucinations, and even death. However, in controlled amounts, it's a lifesaver. Atropine is used as an antidote for poisoning by organophosphate pesticides and nerve agents.

Emergency Medicine: Beyond its role as an antidote, atropine is used in emergency medicine to treat bradycardia (an abnormally slow heart rate) and as a preoperative medication to reduce saliva and bronchial secretions.

Impact on the Nervous System

Blocking the Pathways: Atropine is an anticholinergic agent. This means it blocks the action of the neurotransmitter acetylcholine at its receptors in the nerve synapse. While acetylcholine is essential for the normal functioning of the parasympathetic nervous system, atropine disrupts this, leading to a range of symptoms.

A Cascade of Effects: The blockage of acetylcholine can result in an increased heart rate, decreased salivation, dilation of the pupils, and relaxation of muscles in the respiratory tract. It can also affect the central nervous system, leading to confusion, hallucinations, and at high doses, seizures and respiratory failure.

Case Studies

- **The Soldier's Savior:** During the Gulf War, troops were provided with auto-injectors containing atropine as a countermeasure against potential nerve agent attacks. This highlights the compound's crucial role on modern battlefields.

- **Hallucinogenic Overdoses:** There have been numerous modern-day reports of individuals consuming belladonna or other plants containing atropine, lured by its hallucinogenic properties, only to suffer from severe poisoning.

Atropine's dual nature, both as a potential killer and a lifesaving antidote, is emblematic of the complex interplay between nature, medicine, and human intervention. Its storied history, from the cosmetics of Renaissance ladies to the modern battlefield, underscores the profound impact this compound has had on humanity throughout the ages.

6. Curare: Paralysis from the Amazon

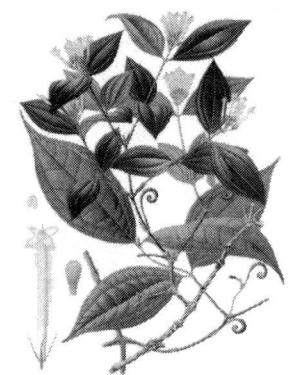

STRYCHNOS TOXIFERA / CURARE

Traditional Uses in Hunting

A Jungle Secret: Nestled deep within the Amazon rainforest, indigenous tribes developed an intricate knowledge of their environment, harnessing the power of the plants around them. Curare, a potent plant-derived poison, emerged as a pivotal tool in their hunting arsenal.

The Blowgun's Companion: Tribesmen would coat the tips of their darts with curare. When shot using a blowgun at prey, the substance would induce paralysis, immobilizing the animal without contaminating its flesh. This ensured that the meat remained safe for consumption.

Preparation and Potency: Creating curare was no simple task. It was typically extracted from plants of the *Menispermaceae* family, notably the *Chondrodendron tomentosum* and *Strychnos toxifera*. The bark and stems of these plants were boiled and reduced to a thick, resinous substance, which was then applied to darts. The potency varied based on the preparation method and specific plant source.

The Silent Assassin

An Ideal Assassin's Tool: Curare's unique mechanism of action made it an ideal poison for those with nefarious intentions. It doesn't actually cause pain or discomfort—victims don't feel themselves being poisoned. Instead, they simply find their muscles refusing to respond, leading to a silent and immobile demise, often mistaken for natural causes.

Difficult to Detect: Historically, one of the reasons curare became a weapon of choice for certain assassins was its difficulty to detect post-mortem. In the absence of specific tests, a curare-induced death could easily be mistaken for a heart failure or other natural causes.

The Case of Dr. Lamson: One of the most notorious instances of curare's use in murder was the case of Dr. George Henry Lamson in the late 19th century. With knowledge of poisons, Dr. Lamson used aconitine and possibly curare to poison his brother-in-law in an attempt to inherit money. While the primary poison was identified as aconitine, curare was rumored to have been a part of his deadly concoctions. The case was notorious not just because of the crime itself but because of Lamson's medical background, which allowed him detailed knowledge of these substances.

Espionage and Rumors: Curare was also rumored to be used by spies and agents during the Cold War. While many of these tales are shrouded in mystery and intrigue, the potency and subtlety of curare made it a frequent topic of speculation in tales of espionage.

Discovery and Adoption in Modern Medicine

From Jungle to Lab: Sir Walter Raleigh is often credited with the first Western account of curare during his expeditions in the late 16th century. However, it wasn't until the 19th and 20th centuries that scientists began to truly understand and harness its properties.

A Surgical Revolution: In the 1930s and 1940s, curare's paralytic properties became of immense interest to the medical community. It was discovered that in controlled doses, curare could relax muscles during surgery, making certain procedures safer and more manageable. This led to the development of synthetic variants which are still in use in modern anesthetics.

Balancing Act: While curare's paralytic properties proved invaluable in surgery, there was a significant risk. An overdose could lead to respiratory failure, and thus, careful dosing and monitoring became essential. With the patient's muscles paralyzed, mechanical ventilation was often necessary to ensure continuous breathing.

Mechanism of Muscle Paralysis

Blocking the Message: Curare's primary action is at the neuromuscular junction, where nerves communicate with muscles. It works by blocking the nicotinic acetylcholine receptors, thereby preventing the neurotransmitter acetylcholine from transmitting signals to muscle fibers.

Resultant Paralysis: Once the signal is blocked, the muscle cannot contract. This results in flaccid paralysis, where muscles become limp and unresponsive. Importantly, this effect is peripheral, meaning it doesn't affect brain function or consciousness. The victim remains aware but immobilized.

Reversal and Recovery: The effects of curare are reversible. In traditional hunting, the paralysis was temporary, allowing tribesmen to reach the immobilized prey before it recovered. In a medical setting, the cessation of curare administration combined with supportive care, like mechanical ventilation, allows the body to metabolize the compound and restore muscle function.

Modern Detection and Forensics

As forensic science progressed, detecting curare in a post-mortem setting became more feasible. Modern toxicology screens, especially when there's suspicion of foul play, can identify even trace amounts of a wide range of substances, including curare.

However, in the past, many potential curare poisonings might have gone unnoticed, with the victims' deaths attributed to natural causes due to the poison's stealthy mode of action. This, combined with the substance's exotic origin, only added to its mystique and dark allure in the annals of crime and poisonings.

Interesting Facts

- **Complex Preparation**: The process of making curare was complex and varied among different indigenous groups. Some recipes required the mixture to be boiled for several days, and the concoction often included a variety of plant species.

- **Specific Plant Sources**: While many plants can produce curare-like compounds, the most potent varieties traditionally came from the genera Strychnos and Chondrodendron. These plants are found in different rainforest regions, suggesting indigenous peoples independently discovered their paralytic properties.

- **Biomedical Research**: Curare and its derivatives have been crucial in understanding how muscles and nerves work. In the 20th century, it was used in research that led to the discovery of neurotransmitters and how nerve signals trigger muscle contractions.

- **Selective Toxicity**: Interestingly, curare is toxic to humans and other mammals, but not to the birds and reptiles commonly hunted with it. This selective toxicity is thought to arise from differences in the nerve receptor structures between these animals and humans.

- **Anaesthetic Revolution**: The introduction of curare into anesthesia in the 1940s by anesthesiologist Harold Griffith greatly improved surgical conditions by providing muscle relaxation without affecting consciousness or pain sensation.

- **Myth and Reality**: There's a myth that a person poisoned with curare could remain conscious until their last breath. However, this is not accurate as the victim would likely pass out due to asphyxia before the end.

- **Historical Impact**: Curare had a significant impact on European colonial forces in South America. They were initially confounded by the natives' ability to kill animals without leaving visible wounds, leading to myths and fears about the "invisible" weapon.

- **Ethnobotanical Knowledge**: The knowledge of curare's preparation was a closely guarded secret among South American tribes. It was often the shaman or a specially trained individual who knew the precise plants and methods to create the paralyzing agent.

- **Antidote Research**: Curare's mode of action has led to research into antidotes that can reverse neuromuscular blockade, which is crucial in cases of accidental poisoning or overdose during medical procedures.

- **Conservation Efforts**: Some of the plant species used to make traditional curare are now threatened due to habitat loss and overharvesting, leading to conservation efforts to preserve both the plants and the indigenous knowledge related to them.

Conclusion

Curare's journey from the depths of the Amazon to the surgical theaters of modern hospitals is a testament to the intertwined destinies of tradition and innovation. It epitomizes the duality of nature's offerings, being both a tool of death and an agent of healing. As we further explore the realm of poisons, curare stands as a beacon, illuminating the delicate balance between harm and hope.

7. Cyanide: A Swift and Silent Killer

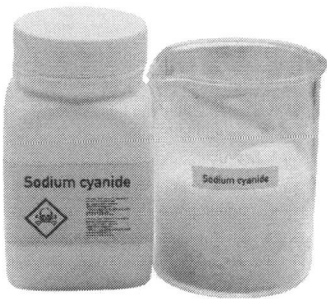

CYANIDE

Nature's Concealed Weapon: The Ubiquity and Subtlety of Cyanide in the Natural World

Cyanogenic Glycosides: These are naturally occurring compounds found in various plants. When cells containing these glycosides are damaged, they can release hydrogen cyanide. It's a defense mechanism against herbivores.

Common Culprits in the Kitchen: Interestingly, several fruits have pits or seeds containing these compounds. Apple seeds, apricot kernels, and cherry pits, among others, carry these substances. While consuming a seed or two is generally harmless to humans due to the small quantity of cyanide, ingesting a significant amount can be harmful.

Defensive Flora: Beyond just fruit seeds, other plants like cassava, flax, and certain species of bamboo also possess cyanogenic glycosides. For some of these plants, especially cassava, proper processing and cooking are vital to reduce the toxic content.

Adaptive Evolution: It's believed that this trait evolved as a defense mechanism against grazing animals. An animal consuming large quantities of these plants might experience toxic effects, deterring it from further consumption.

Alchemy of the Modern Age: Crafting Cyanide in Contemporary Labs

The Andrussow Process: This is the most common industrial method of producing hydrogen cyanide (HCN). It involves the direct oxidation of methane and ammonia over a platinum catalyst at temperatures exceeding 1200°C. The process is efficient and favored because it uses relatively cheap raw materials.

Other Synthetic Methods: The Shawinigan Process, an older method, involves the electrochemical reduction of atmospheric nitrogen in an aqueous solution of an alkali metal cyanide. Another method, the Degussa process, produces HCN by reacting formamide with oxygen.

Quality and Purity: The demands of certain industries, especially those related to food and pharmaceuticals, require hydrogen cyanide of high purity. Advanced purification methods have been developed to meet these stringent standards.

Industrial Uses: The Duality of Cyanide's Applications

Mining Endeavors: Cyanide's ability to bond with precious metals like gold and silver makes it invaluable in the mining industry. The gold cyanidation process involves treating ore with a cyanide solution, which bonds with the gold, allowing it to be separated from other materials.

Electroplating and Beyond: In the realm of metallurgy, cyanide is used for electroplating metals like gold and silver onto other objects. This process provides a decorative finish or a protective coating.

Chemical Synthesis: The chemical industry employs cyanide in the production of various organic compounds, some of which are precursors to valuable products like pharmaceuticals, dyes, and plastics.

From the unsuspecting fruit bowl to the state-of-the-art industrial plant, cyanide's presence and significance in our world are undeniable. Its dual nature—as both a life-taking poison and a life-enhancing tool—remains a testament to the complex interplay between nature and human ingenuity.

Understanding the Deadly Mechanism

Assault on Cellular Respiration: The Intricacies of Cyanide's Attack

The Mitochondrial Electron Transport Chain: The mitochondria in our cells can be likened to powerhouses, producing energy in the form of adenosine triphosphate (ATP). Central to this process is the electron transport chain, a series of protein complexes located within the mitochondrial membrane.

Cyanide's Target: Cyanide specifically targets cytochrome c oxidase, also known as Complex IV, one of the essential proteins in the electron transport chain. By binding to this protein, cyanide stops the final step of electron transport, preventing the transfer of electrons to oxygen. This binding is almost irreversible, making cyanide's effects particularly potent.

Energy Deprivation: As a result of the halting of the electron transport chain, cells can no longer produce the ATP they require. This ATP deprivation quickly affects organs with high energy demands, such as the brain and the heart.

System-wide Shutdown: From Molecular Blockage to Full-Body Crisis

Brain Dysfunction: The brain is one of the organs most sensitive to changes in oxygen and ATP levels. A drop in ATP production can lead to neurological symptoms like confusion, dizziness, and seizures.

Cardiac Complications: The heart, reliant on a steady supply of ATP, can experience decreased contractility. This leads to symptoms such as arrhythmias, low blood pressure, and ultimately cardiac arrest.

Respiratory Distress: Since oxygen can no longer be effectively utilized in cells, the body responds by trying to increase oxygen intake. This can lead to rapid breathing or even gasping for air, a tell-tale sign of cyanide poisoning.

Counteraction and Treatment: Racing Against Time

Mechanism of Antidotes: Hydroxocobalamin, one of the primary antidotes, acts as a cyanide sponge. It binds to the cyanide molecules, forming cyanocobalamin (Vitamin B12) which is less toxic and is excreted in urine.

Swift Administration is Crucial: Given the rapid and devastating effects of cyanide, time is of the essence. Administering the antidote within minutes can be the difference between life and death.

Supportive Care: Alongside specific antidote treatment, patients often require supportive care. This can include oxygen therapy to counteract the hypoxia and medications to support blood pressure and heart function.

The detailed interaction between cyanide and our body's cellular machinery highlights the precision with which nature operates — and how a single molecule, when out of place, can wreak havoc on an intricate system.

Infamous Cyanide Poisoning Cases

The Jonestown Massacre: A Chilling Tale of Devotion and Despair

> **Background**: Located in Guyana, Jonestown was established as a remote settlement by the Peoples Temple, a cult led by Jim Jones. Portrayed as a socialist paradise and a haven from the perceived evils of the outside world, it instead became the site of one of history's most tragic mass suicides.
>
> **The Deadly Drink**: On November 18, 1978, under Jones's directive, a deadly concoction of cyanide, sedatives, and flavored drink mix (often mistaken as Kool-Aid) was prepared. Parents administered the poison to their children before consuming it themselves.
>
> **Aftermath**: The world was shocked as images emerged of hundreds of bodies scattered across the settlement. Investigations revealed tales of manipulation, abuse, and coercion within the cult. The Jonestown Massacre serves as a grim reminder of the dangers of blind allegiance and the depths of human susceptibility.

Tylenol Murders: The Crisis that Changed Consumer Safety

Initial Shock: Between September 29 and October 1, 1982, seven individuals in the Chicago area unknowingly took Extra-Strength Tylenol capsules laced with a lethal dose of cyanide. All seven died rapidly after ingestion.

Investigation and Implications: While law enforcement, with the help of the manufacturer Johnson & Johnson, launched an extensive investigation, the culprit was never definitively identified. The murders had a profound impact on consumer safety and trust.

Legacy: These events led to significant changes in the packaging of over-the-counter and consumable products, with tamper-evident seals becoming standard. It spurred the pharmaceutical industry and lawmakers to prioritize consumer safety, leading to the introduction of the federal Anti-Tampering Act in 1983.

Hitler's Inner Circle: Desperate Acts in the Face of Defeat

The Bunker: By 1945, as the Allied forces rapidly approached, Hitler and his closest associates took refuge in the Führerbunker, an underground shelter in Berlin.

The Final Moments: While the exact circumstances of Hitler's death are shrouded in mystery and controversy, it is more definitively believed that many of his associates, seeing no way out and fearing capture, turned to cyanide as a means of suicide. Eva Braun, Hitler's longtime companion and short-lived wife, is believed to have taken cyanide alongside him.

Symbolism: The mass suicides within Hitler's inner circle symbolized the collapse of the Third Reich. The choice of cyanide, easily concealed in breakable capsules, showcased the level of preparation and forethought some had given to their potential end.

These cases, though vastly different in context, underline cyanide's potency and its enduring, dark appeal in moments of desperation, manipulation, and malice.

Cyanide has played a role in various high-profile poisoning cases and assassination attempts throughout history due to its potency and rapid-acting nature. Here are a few more cases involving the use of cyanide:

Alan Chmurny: In a more recent case from the early 2000s, Maryland resident Alan Chmurny was accused of poisoning his co-worker's drink with mercury(II) nitrate. When found guilty and faced with a long prison sentence, Chmurny committed suicide in his jail cell using cyanide.

Grigori Rasputin's Alleged Assassination Attempt: While the full truth behind Rasputin's death is shrouded in mystery, one popular version claims that Prince Felix Yusupov and other conspirators first tried to kill Rasputin by feeding him wine and pastries laced with cyanide. According to this account, the poison seemingly failed, leading to subsequent assassination attempts that night.

The Tokyo Subway Sarin Attack: While this 1995 event orchestrated by the Aum Shinrikyo cult primarily involved the nerve agent sarin, there were previous instances where the cult used cyanide. They attempted to release hydrogen cyanide in several Tokyo subway stations but were unsuccessful in causing mass casualties.

Michael Swango: An American serial killer and former licensed medical professional, Swango is believed to have caused up to 60 deaths and illnesses of patients and colleagues, using various means, including injecting cyanide.

Mass Suicide in Temirtau, Kazakhstan: In 1987, 53 members of a spiritual group committed mass suicide in Kazakhstan. The group, following a charismatic leader, believed that they would be reborn on another planet. They consumed cyanide mixed with water.

Bangladesh Cyanide Sweets Poisoning: In 1988, over 70 people died after consuming toxic paracetamol syrup, later found to be contaminated with diethylene glycol. In the aftermath, there was public fear and suspicion of medicine. Exploiting this fear, an individual poisoned sweets with cyanide, leading to several deaths.

Cyanide's easy accessibility, its swift action, and the difficulty in detecting it (especially in earlier times) made it a favored choice for many crimes, assassination attempts, and suicides. The notorious nature of these cases has also imprinted the poison deeply in public consciousness.

Interesting Facts

- **Historical Uses**: Beyond its modern notoriety, cyanide has historical roots. Ancient Romans, for instance, are believed to have used cyanide salts derived from peach and cherry pits in poison-laden rings intended for political assassinations.

- **Smell of Almonds**: One of the distinctive characteristics of cyanide, especially hydrogen cyanide, is its bitter almond smell. However, not everyone can detect this aroma. The ability to smell cyanide is based on genetics, with a significant portion of the population being unable to identify the scent.

- **Cyanide in Space**: Interstellar space contains vast clouds of hydrogen cyanide. Astronomers believe these clouds play a vital role in the formation of amino acids, which are the building blocks of proteins essential for life.

- **Cassava and Cyanide**: The cassava root, a staple food for millions, especially in Africa and South America, naturally contains cyanogenic glycosides which release hydrogen cyanide when the plant tissue is damaged. However, when prepared correctly (soaked, dried, and cooked), the cyanide levels are diminished, making the root safe to eat.

- **Smoke Inhalation**: One of the dangers of house fires isn't just the fire itself, but the release of toxic gases. Many synthetic materials, when burned, release hydrogen cyanide. This makes smoke inhalation during house fires particularly dangerous.

- **Laetrile and Pseudo-science**: In the 1970s, a compound named Laetrile, which breaks down into cyanide, was widely promoted as an alternative cancer cure. However, no scientific evidence supports this claim, and its usage can be harmful due to the cyanide it releases.

- **Use in Gold Mining**: The gold mining industry uses cyanide to separate gold from ore, a process called gold cyanidation. The gold binds to the cyanide, forming a soluble compound that can be separated from the waste. The cyanide is then removed from the gold, and the gold is refined further.

- **Environmental Impact**: Cyanide can have devastating effects on the environment if not managed properly, especially in mining operations. Fish are particularly sensitive to cyanide. Many governments regulate the disposal of cyanide to protect aquatic life and water supplies.

- **Therapeutic Use**: Despite its toxicity, there's research into the potential therapeutic uses of cyanide. In incredibly low doses, it might have applications in treating certain diseases, but research is in the preliminary stages.

- **Quick vs. Slow Poisoning**: While cyanide is famous for acting swiftly, prolonged exposure to lower doses can lead to symptoms like weakness, confusion, excessive sleepiness, headache, and even coma, making diagnosis challenging in cases of chronic exposure.

In understanding cyanide, it's clear that context is crucial. In one setting, it's a deadly poison; in another, it's a crucial industrial tool or even a potential medicine. This duality is a hallmark of many chemicals, but few have captured the popular imagination quite like cyanide.

8. Digitalis: Nature's Heart-stopping Toxin

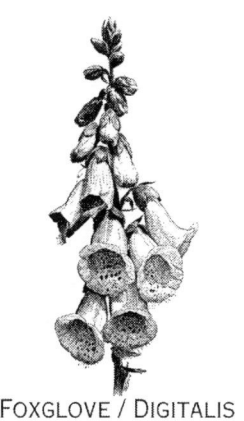

FOXGLOVE / DIGITALIS

The Deadly Beauty of Foxgloves

A Vibrant Facade: The foxglove (Digitalis purpurea) is one of the most iconic plants found in gardens across Europe and North America. Tall and statuesque, its vibrant tubular flowers are bell-shaped and hang down in an elegant droop. These flowers can range from deep purple with speckled throats to soft pink and pristine white. While they're an aesthetic delight for gardeners and flower enthusiasts, the beauty of the foxglove conceals a dangerous secret.

Botanical Profile: The foxglove is a biennial plant, which means it completes its life cycle in two years. In its first year, it produces a tight rosette of leaves close to the ground. By the second year, it shoots up a tall stem adorned with its iconic bell-shaped flowers. The leaves are large, veiny, and have a slightly downy texture, and they contain a majority of the plant's toxic compounds.

Toxin Throughout: While the flowers of the foxglove are often the most admired, every part of the plant – from the roots to the seeds – contains the deadly cardiac glycosides, particularly digitoxin and digoxin. Even the water in a vase holding foxglove flowers can have traces of the toxin.

Extraction: Historically, if someone wanted to extract the poisonous compounds from foxgloves, they would typically dry and crush the leaves. This would be followed by an extraction process using organic solvents like alcohol. The resulting concoction would be concentrated and could be administered in various forms. It's crucial to note that this method is imprecise and extremely dangerous, as the line between a therapeutic dose and a lethal one is razor-thin. In modern times, pharmaceutical processes to extract digoxin are more sophisticated and precise, ensuring the right concentration for medicinal purposes.

Nature's Warning and Folklore: Foxgloves have inspired numerous legends and tales, which perhaps serve as a testament to their potent nature. In certain traditions, they're believed to be the favored flowers of fairies. The name "foxglove" itself is believed to be a distortion of "folk's glove," alluding to the fairy folk. Legends in some regions warned against picking or harming the plant, lest one draws the ire of its supernatural guardians.

When writing about the extraction, it's essential to approach with caution and emphasize that this is a historical perspective. Modern extraction for medicinal purposes is conducted under strict regulations and with advanced equipment to ensure patient safety. The process described above is not meant as a guide but rather a historical perspective on how this plant's toxins might have been accessed in earlier times.

Historical Medicinal Uses and Dangers

A Legacy in Ancient Medicine: The medicinal qualities of the foxglove, while prevalent in European traditions, can trace their origins further back. Ancient Roman physicians, such as Pliny the Elder, referenced the plant in their writings, highlighting its potency and potential dangers. Pliny described it as a powerful diuretic, which the Romans used to treat what they termed "dropsy" - an archaic term for edema or the accumulation of fluid in the body.

Medieval Mysticism and Medicine: In medieval times, foxglove was sometimes used in folk medicine as both a remedy and a poison. Given its striking appearance, it also featured in various mystical and magical preparations. Herbalists of the era held a deep respect for the plant due to its dual nature – it could both heal and harm.

Withering's Pioneering Work: Dr. William Withering's discovery in the 18th century marked a significant turning point. He came across the plant's therapeutic potential somewhat by chance, when he learned of an old woman's herbal remedy for dropsy that had a notable success rate. Intrigued, Withering undertook a decade-long study, eventually isolating foxglove as the active ingredient in the remedy. In 1785, he published "An Account of the Foxglove," detailing 156 case studies and emphasizing the plant's utility in treating heart failure.

The Therapeutic Paradox: Withering's work highlighted the paradox of foxglove: its capacity to both alleviate heart conditions and induce fatal ones. He was acutely aware of the narrow therapeutic window and wrote extensively about dosage, preparation, and potential side effects. This "window" meant that just a slight overdose could lead to deadly consequences. Symptoms of an overdose included nausea, vomiting, hallucinations, and a potentially fatal slowing of the heart.

Victorian Era and Accidental Poisonings: As the Victorian era saw a surge in self-medication and the use of home remedies, there were several documented cases of foxglove poisoning. Often, it was mistaken for other benign herbs or was misused due to a lack of standardized dosing guidelines. These instances further underscored the need for precise dosing and professional oversight when using such potent substances.

From Deadly Herb to Lifesaving Drug: Despite its tumultuous history, the compounds derived from foxglove, particularly digoxin, became staples in modern cardiology. They're used to treat various heart conditions, such as atrial fibrillation and heart failure. Modern pharmaceutical methods allow for the precise extraction and dosing of these compounds, minimizing the risks that historically accompanied the use of foxglove.

How Digitalis Affects the Heart

Deep Dive into Cardiac Glycosides: The foxglove plant is a rich source of potent compounds called cardiac glycosides, primarily digitoxin and digoxin. These molecules have a unique mechanism of action, targeting cellular machinery that's crucial for heart function.

Inhibition of the Sodium-Potassium Pump: At the cellular level, cardiac glycosides primarily act by inhibiting the sodium-potassium ATPase pump. This pump actively transports sodium out of cells and potassium into cells. By inhibiting this pump, digitalis increases the sodium concentration inside the cells.

Calcium's Central Role: The rise in intracellular sodium indirectly leads to an increase in intracellular calcium. This is because the sodium-calcium exchanger, which typically pumps calcium out of the cell in exchange for sodium, becomes less effective. As a result, more calcium stays within the cells.

Strength in Contraction: High levels of calcium in heart cells enhance the force of myocardial contraction. In layman's terms, it makes the heart squeeze more powerfully. This can be beneficial in certain conditions where the heart is failing to pump blood effectively, such as congestive heart failure.

The Tightrope of Therapeutics: The very quality that makes cardiac glycosides therapeutic — their ability to strengthen heart contractions — can also make them dangerous. Overstimulation of the heart can result in arrhythmias. These irregular heart rhythms can range from benign extra beats to life-threatening conditions such as ventricular fibrillation.

Symptoms of Digitalis Toxicity: Beyond arrhythmias, digitalis poisoning can present a myriad of symptoms. Patients might experience gastrointestinal disturbances like nausea, vomiting, and diarrhea. Neurological signs include confusion, drowsiness, and even hallucinations. One particularly characteristic symptom of digitalis toxicity is xanthopsia, where vision takes on a yellow tint.

Modern Utilization and Monitoring: While raw foxglove extracts have fallen out of favor, digitoxin and especially digoxin remain important tools in the cardiologist's arsenal. They're primarily used for atrial fibrillation, a common type of arrhythmia, and heart failure. Given the narrow therapeutic window, patients on these drugs often undergo regular blood tests to ensure that levels remain within the safe and effective range.

Digitalis, due to its potency and narrow therapeutic window, has been implicated in a number of noteworthy poisonings, both accidental and intentional:

Agatha Christie's Mysteries: The renowned crime fiction author, Agatha Christie, used poison, including digitalis, in many of her novels. One of the most famous is *The Murder of Roger Ackroyd*, where the victim's wife dies from an overdose of medication containing digitalis. Christie's accurate portrayal of the symptoms of digitalis poisoning reflects her background as a pharmacy assistant during World War I.

Dr. Michael Swango: A licensed medical professional turned serial killer, Dr. Swango is believed to have caused the deaths of up to 60 patients and colleagues over 17 years. Among the substances he used to poison his victims was digoxin, a derivative of digitalis.

Yushchenko Poisoning: Though the primary agent used in the poisoning of Viktor Yushchenko, the former President of Ukraine, was dioxin, some sources speculated on the presence of digitalis, given some of the symptoms he exhibited. However, this claim remains unsubstantiated.

Accidental Overdoses: Given the thin line between therapeutic and toxic doses, there have been numerous recorded cases of patients accidentally overdosing on medications containing digitalis. These instances underscore the importance of precise dosing and regular monitoring for patients prescribed this drug.

Murder in Australia: In 2002, a woman was convicted in Australia for the murder of her partner using digitalis. Her crime was discovered when an autopsy revealed elevated levels of the toxin in the victim's blood.

Historical Use: In earlier centuries, when the difference between therapeutic and lethal doses was less understood, there were undoubtedly many unrecorded or misattributed deaths due to digitalis. It's worth noting that digitalis preparations would vary in strength depending on their source and preparation, making it even trickier to dose correctly.

These instances highlight the double-edged sword that is digitalis. In the right hands and at the correct dose, it's a life-saving medicine. However, its potency and the fine line between therapeutic and toxic doses have also made it a tool for malevolent intent.

Interesting facts

- **Name Origin**: The name "foxglove" is believed to have derived from the term "folk's glove." The "folk" referred to are possibly fairies, and the plant's flowers resemble the fingers of a glove. Some legends even suggest that fairies gave the flowers to foxes to wear as gloves, so they wouldn't be heard while raiding chicken coops!

- **Van Gogh's Yellow Vision**: The post-impressionist painter Vincent van Gogh was known to take digitalis for epilepsy. Some art historians speculate that the yellow-dominated palette of some of his later works, including the famous "Starry Night," might have been influenced by xanthopsia, a side effect of digitalis toxicity that causes a yellow tint to the vision.

- **Diverse Medical Use**: Apart from heart-related ailments, digitalis was historically used for a variety of conditions, including tuberculosis, fevers, and even insanity.

- **Plant Varieties**: While the purple foxglove (Digitalis purpurea) is the most well-known, there are other species like the straw foxglove (Digitalis lutea) and the large yellow foxglove (Digitalis grandiflora). Each has its own unique appearance, but all contain the potent cardiac glycosides.

- **Digitalis in the Garden**: Despite its toxic properties, foxglove is a popular ornamental plant in many gardens. It's valued for its tall, spike-like clusters of tubular flowers that attract pollinators. However, gardeners with children or pets often exercise caution or avoid planting it due to its toxicity.

- **Digitalis Resistance**: Some animals have developed a resistance to digitalis. For example, the caterpillar of the foxglove pug moth feeds on the leaves of the plant without any ill effect. Similarly, snails can eat foxglove leaves and store the toxin in their bodies, making them unpalatable to predators.

- **Modern Medicine Precautions**: Today, patients prescribed digitalis-derived medications typically receive regular blood tests to ensure they remain within the therapeutic range. This tight monitoring helps prevent unintentional overdoses.

This fascinating blend of history, culture, science, and legend underscores how digitalis, like many natural substances, can be both a boon and a bane. It serves as a potent reminder of the power of nature and the respect it commands.

9. Hemlock: The Poison of Philosophers

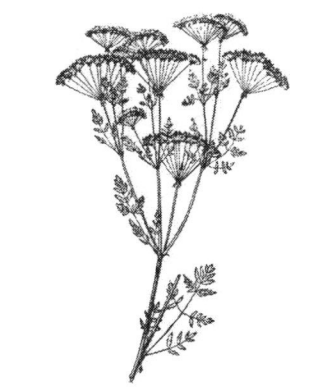

CONIUM MACULATUM / HEMLOCK

Its Ancient History and Ties to Socrates

Socrates' Philosophical End: The story of Socrates' death not only provides a historical account of hemlock's lethal reputation but also offers a profound look into the philosophical attitudes of the time towards death and the law. Conium maculatum's lethal brew, in this context, was not just a method of execution but a tool for delivering a statement about dignity and wisdom in the face of an unjust death. Socrates, rather than fleeing or protesting his innocence, chose to comply with the sentence. By drinking the hemlock, he turned his death into a final teaching moment about the soul's immortality and virtue, topics that still resonate through the philosophical discourse to this day.

Hemlock in the Courtroom: In ancient Athens, hemlock was the state-sanctioned method of execution for condemned prisoners. Its selection was partly due to the symptoms of its poisoning being less gruesome and more controlled compared to other methods of the time. The preparation of the hemlock potion was a solemn ritual, with the condemned allowed to pray before consuming the fatal concoction. It is said that the state provided a significant amount of the poison to ensure a quick and certain death, reflecting the society's approach to death as a civic and ritualistic duty.

Sacred and Profane Associations: Hemlock's connection to Hecate and Cerberus conjures images of a plant that is both sacred and profane, a botanical paradox that can guide souls to the afterlife or be wielded as a weapon against life. This mythological backdrop adds a layer of divine fatalism to the use of hemlock, suggesting that its ingestion might have been seen not just as a punishment but as an ordained passage decreed by the gods.

Medicinal Juxtaposition: The dual nature of hemlock—its ability to take life and its capacity to ease pain—reflects the broader historical perspective on poisons and medicine. In the hands of the skilled, such as the physicians of old, hemlock's extracts were measured and administered to exploit its analgesic properties.

Yet an error in dosage could turn a cure into a death sentence. This balance has fascinated medical practitioners for centuries and has made hemlock a subject of study in the evolution of pharmacology, where the line between remedy and poison has always been razor-thin.

Symbolic Legacy: Hemlock's infamous use in the death of Socrates has left a lasting mark on cultural and philosophical symbolism. It represents the ultimate sacrifice for one's principles and the concept that the search for truth may lead to deadly consequences. It is emblematic of the ancient philosophical stance where the pursuit of knowledge and adherence to personal and civic virtue were deemed worth facing death.

Through these expanded details, hemlock is seen not only as a mere plant or poison but also as an emblematic agent in human history and culture, carrying with it stories of death, philosophy, and the eternal human quest to balance the powers of life and death.

Physical Properties and Symptoms

Deceptive Aesthetics: Hemlock's physical traits could easily lead to its mistaken identification for a non-toxic plant, which historically has resulted in accidental poisonings. Its tall stature and delicate, fern-like foliage lend it an elegance that belies its lethal nature. The purple or red blemishes on its stem were once thought to be a warning sign provided by nature, marking the plant with a visual cue of its toxicity, as if stained by the blood of its victims.

Toxic Components: The plant's notorious toxicity comes from a variety of alkaloids, primarily coniine, which has a chemical structure similar to nicotine and is similarly neurotoxic. These compounds are concentrated in the seeds and roots but are present throughout the plant, with toxicity remaining potent even when the plant is dried.

Insidious Onset: Upon ingestion, the poison's onset is deceptively gentle, initially producing symptoms akin to drunkenness or lightheadedness. This may lure the poisoned individual into a false sense of security before the more severe symptoms manifest.

Systematic Paralysis: The alkaloids in hemlock are neuromuscular blocking agents, which leads to a sequence of symptoms that start with numbness in the extremities and progress to full muscular paralysis. Notably, the mind remains clear and alert, a particularly cruel aspect of the poison, as the victim is aware of their gradual, inexorable descent into paralysis.

The Final Phase: The final symptoms are a terrifying cascade: The muscles responsible for breathing begin to fail, and the victim experiences the horror of asphyxia while fully conscious. The heart continues to beat until the very end, as it is not directly affected by the toxins, meaning death comes solely from the inability to breathe.

Historical Accounts: Detailed descriptions of hemlock poisoning, such as those provided by the accounts of Socrates' death, have been invaluable for toxicologists and historians. They provide insight not only into the progression of symptoms but also into the demeanor with which individuals faced the effects of the poison, offering a window into ancient practices of execution and societal views on death and dignity.

In expanding on the physical properties and symptoms of hemlock, we get a picture of a poison that is swift and merciless, one that has claimed its place in history not just for its deadliness but also for the philosophical and cultural implications surrounding its use.

How Hemlock Disrupts Biological Systems

Targeting the Nervous System: Coniine, the primary alkaloid toxin found in hemlock, is a potent neurotoxin that mimics the structure of neurotransmitter molecules. It binds to the nicotinic acetylcholine receptors at the neuromuscular junction – the critical point where nerve impulses are transmitted to muscles.

Molecular Mimicry and Disruption: By binding to these receptors, coniine effectively blocks the action of acetylcholine, a neurotransmitter that is essential for muscle contraction. Normally, when acetylcholine binds to its receptor, it induces a change that triggers muscle contraction. Coniine's interference prevents this process, leading to a breakdown in communication between the nerves and muscles.

A Cascade of Paralysis: As a result of this blockage, voluntary muscle contractions become impossible, initiating with the smaller, more distal muscles of the body and then spreading to the larger, proximal muscle groups. The diaphragm and intercostal muscles, crucial for breathing, are among the last to be affected, leading to respiratory failure.

Deceptive Recovery and Relapse: Interestingly, there may be a period where the victim seems to recover, as the body metabolically processes the coniine. However, if a lethal dose has been ingested, the respite is temporary. Often, the toxin concentration is too overwhelming for the liver and kidneys to clear, leading to a relapse into paralysis.

No Antidote: While there are treatments that can support the body during hemlock poisoning, such as artificial respiration, there is no antidote that can reverse the effects of the toxins once they have bound to acetylcholine receptors. This renders the poisoning particularly dangerous and often fatal without immediate medical intervention.

Irreversible Damage: In cases of severe poisoning, even if the victim survives, there may be long-term or permanent damage to the central nervous system due to the prolonged lack of oxygen and potential buildup of toxins that can affect the brain.

In its essence, hemlock's lethality is a direct result of its ability to bring the body's communication with its muscles to a complete standstill, embodying the paradox of nature's capacity to sustain life and also to silently extinguish it. Its indelible mark on human history, medicine, and culture endures, a perpetual symbol of the thin line between remedy and poison.

Cases Through History

Hemlock poisoning cases beyond the historical account of Socrates are not as commonly documented in ancient texts, but there have been instances throughout history where hemlock has been implicated:

> **Medieval Trials and Executions**: In medieval Europe, hemlock was sometimes used as a means of execution. It was chosen for its relative 'humane' aspect of inducing death without physical pain, as the victim would become numb and lose consciousness before dying.
>
> **Accidental Poisonings**: There have been numerous reports of accidental poisonings throughout history, often due to the misidentification of the plant. Hemlock can be mistaken for edible plants such as wild carrots or parsley.

Medicinal Misadventures: Due to its medicinal properties when used in small doses, hemlock was also occasionally responsible for accidental poisonings when it was incorrectly prepared or administered in too high a dose.

Suicide: Like other poisons, hemlock has been used for suicide, with some historical figures allegedly choosing it to control their death. However, specific names and details often remain unverified.

Assassinations and Murders: There are accounts of hemlock being used for murder, but many of these are not well-documented or are from unverifiable sources. In many historical contexts, poisoning was often a method of assassination due to its discreet nature.

Modern Cases: In modern times, cases of hemlock poisoning are rare but have occurred, often due to misidentification by foragers. For example, in 2002, a group in Scotland accidentally consumed hemlock water dropwort, a plant with similar toxic properties, mistaking it for an edible herb.

Folk Medicine Misapplications: There are also scattered reports from the 19th and early 20th centuries of hemlock being used in folk remedies that resulted in overdoses, as the practice of medicine was not as regulated as it is today.

While hemlock poisoning is not as common as other forms of toxicological emergencies in the modern era, these historical and more recent cases illustrate the ongoing risks associated with toxic plants. They underscore the importance of education about plant identification and the dangers of using wild plants without thorough knowledge.

Interesting Facts

- **Name Origin**: The name "hemlock" is believed to derive from the Old English "hemlic," "henleac," or similar variations, which possibly relate to the plant's hem-like odor (resembling that of the bird) or perhaps from "healm," meaning "straw," due to its hollow stems.

- **Toxicity Variability**: The level of toxicity in hemlock can vary depending on several factors, including the season, the plant's growth phase, and geographical conditions. It's usually most toxic during the early stages of growth in the spring.

- **Historical Medicinal Use**: Despite its toxicity, hemlock was used in traditional medicine to treat conditions like tumors, ulcers, and rheumatism. It was administered in very small doses, and practitioners needed to be careful to avoid toxic effects.

- **Linnaeus's Interest**: Carl Linnaeus, the father of modern taxonomy, was so fascinated by hemlock that he experimented on himself by taking small doses of the plant to understand its effects.

- **Socrates' Philosophical Stance**: It's worth noting that Socrates had the option to escape his death sentence but chose to consume the hemlock as a statement of his philosophical beliefs, emphasizing the importance of the rule of law.

- **Detective Literature**: Hemlock has been featured in detective novels and murder mysteries as a classic means of a seemingly untraceable assassination, owing to its natural origin and historical notoriety.

- **Identification Difficulty**: Hemlock's resemblance to non-toxic plants has been the cause of accidental poisonings, as it's easily confused with wild carrot (Daucus carota), parsnip, or parsley, which are harmless and often foraged.

- **Pesticide Resistance**: Interestingly, there have been reports in the agricultural world of hemlock being resistant to common pesticides, making it a tough weed to control in areas where it is considered invasive.

- **Shakespeare's Reference**: In Shakespeare's play "Macbeth," the witches' brew contains "slips of yew silvered in the moon's eclipse," which some scholars believe refers to hemlock, tying the plant to witchcraft and dark rituals.

- **Alkaloid Research**: The study of the alkaloids in hemlock, particularly coniine, has contributed to the field of organic chemistry and has helped in understanding the structure and function of neurotoxic alkaloids.

- **Wildlife and Livestock Risks**: Hemlock is not only toxic to humans but also to animals. Livestock poisonings occur when animals accidentally consume the plant, which can lead to significant losses in farming communities.

- **Survival Stories**: There have been rare cases where victims of hemlock poisoning survived after ingesting small amounts and receiving prompt medical treatment, which usually involves supportive care since there's no specific antidote for hemlock toxicity.

The duality of hemlock as both a historically significant plant and a deadly poison continues to captivate both the scientific community and popular culture, adding layers to its dark legacy.

10. Mercury: The Mad Hatter's Nemesis

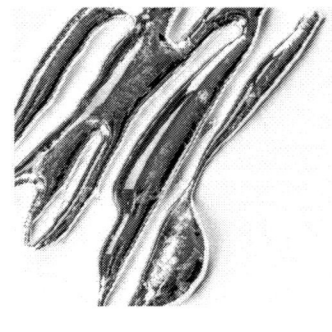

MURCURY

Historical Uses in Medicine and Cosmetics

Medicinal Applications: A Double-Edged Sword

Ancient Practices: The use of mercury in medicine dates back to ancient civilizations. The Greeks, for example, used mercury in ointments for skin diseases and wounds, while the Romans included it in various medicinal concoctions for a range of ailments.

Ayurveda and Traditional Chinese Medicine: In Ayurvedic medicine, mercury was used in small amounts in certain formulations, believed to treat digestive issues and chronic diseases. Similarly, traditional Chinese medicine utilized mercury in its elemental form and as cinnabar (mercury sulfide) for purported life-extending and rejuvenating properties.

Syphilis Treatment: One of the most well-known historical uses of mercury was in treating syphilis, a prevalent and dreaded sexually transmitted disease in the 16th and 17th centuries. Mercury was administered through various methods, including topically as an ointment, orally, and even through fumigation, where patients were exposed to mercury vapors. While some patients experienced temporary relief, the toxic side effects, such as severe mouth ulcers, tooth loss, and neurological damage, were often as debilitating as the disease itself.

Cosmetic Use: Beauty at a Cost

Ancient Egyptian Cosmetics: The use of mercury-based compounds in cosmetics has roots in ancient Egypt. Cinnabar was prized for its vibrant red color, used in cosmetics for coloring lips and cheeks. This practice highlighted the societal value placed on appearance and beauty, even at potential health costs.

Skin Lightening in Europe: In the 18th century, European women used creams containing mercury to lighten their skin, a beauty trend driven by the association of pale skin with nobility and upper-class status. Unaware of the toxic effects, long-term users of these creams often suffered from skin damage, weakened teeth, and other health issues related to mercury exposure.

Cultural and Social Implications: These practices reflect the historical cultural norms where beauty standards often overrode awareness of potential health risks. The use of mercury in cosmetics underscores the lengths to which people have gone to conform to these beauty ideals.

Amalgams and Dentistry: A Controversial Legacy

Introduction of Dental Amalgams: Mercury's use in dentistry began in the 19th century with the development of dental amalgams. These amalgams, a mixture of mercury with other metals like silver and tin, provided a durable and malleable material for filling cavities.

Advantages and Drawbacks: The use of amalgams revolutionized dental care due to their ease of application and durability compared to previous filling materials. However, the potential health risks associated with mercury exposure led to controversy and debate within the dental community and among the public.

Modern Shifts in Dentistry: With the rise of health and environmental concerns, many countries have reduced or restricted the use of mercury in dentistry. This shift has been accompanied by the development of alternative filling materials, such as composite resins and ceramics, which are safer and aesthetically more pleasing.

In summary, mercury's historical usage in medicine, cosmetics, and dentistry illustrates a complex interplay between perceived benefits and the gradual recognition of its toxic effects. This history underscores the evolving understanding of medical and cosmetic practices and the importance of prioritizing health and safety in these fields.

Notable Mercury Poisoning Incidents

Minamata Disease: A Tragic Environmental Disaster

Devastating Industrial Impact: The Minamata Disease incident, one of the most catastrophic cases of industrial pollution, began in the 1950s when a chemical factory released methylmercury into Minamata Bay, Japan. This toxic substance bioaccumulated in fish and shellfish, a staple in the diet of the local communities.

Severe Health Consequences: People who consumed the contaminated seafood developed severe neurological symptoms, including numbness in the hands and feet, muscle weakness, damage to hearing and speech, and in extreme cases, paralysis and death. Pregnant women who ate the contaminated fish gave birth to infants with severe developmental disabilities, known as congenital Minamata Disease.

International Attention and Aftermath: The Minamata incident brought worldwide attention to the dangers of industrial pollution and the need for strict environmental regulations. It led to significant changes in policies regarding industrial waste management and environmental protection in Japan and around the world.

Hatters' Disease: The Cost of Fashion

Industrial Hazard in Hat-Making: During the 18th to 20th centuries, mercury nitrate was used in the process of curing felt used in hat-making. The prolonged exposure to mercury vapors in poorly ventilated workshops led to the accumulation of mercury in the bodies of the hat-makers.

Symptoms and Social Impact: Workers developed a range of symptoms, now collectively known as Mad Hatter's Disease or erethism mercurialis. These included tremors (hence the term "hatter's shakes"), emotional instability, personality changes, and hallucinations. The phrase "mad as a hatter" became popular in the 19th century, reflecting the prevalence of these symptoms among hat-makers.

Regulatory Changes: This occupational hazard eventually led to changes in industrial practices and the decline in the use of mercury in the hat-making industry, particularly as awareness of the health risks grew and alternative processes were developed.

Newark Bay Incident: A Modern Cautionary Tale

Mercury in the Waterways: In the late 20th century, the Newark Bay Complex in New Jersey was found to be heavily contaminated with mercury, a result of decades of industrial activity in the region.

Environmental and Health Implications: High levels of mercury in the bay led to the contamination of fish and other aquatic life, posing serious health risks to people who consumed these species. This prompted a ban on fishing, affecting the livelihoods of local fishermen and the food supply of the community.

Remediation Efforts: The discovery led to extensive cleanup and remediation efforts, as well as stricter environmental monitoring and regulations to prevent such incidents in the future. The Newark Bay incident serves as a reminder of the long-term environmental and health consequences of industrial pollution.

These incidents underscore the widespread impact of mercury poisoning, affecting not only individual health but also communities and ecosystems. They highlight the need for vigilance, responsible industrial practices, and effective environmental regulation to prevent such tragedies.

Interesting Facts:

- **Liquid Metal**: Mercury is the only metal that is liquid at standard room temperature and pressure. Its melting point is -38.83 degrees Celsius (-37.89 degrees Fahrenheit), which makes it uniquely liquid in a range from that low temperature up to its boiling point.

- **Alchemical Symbolism**: In alchemy, mercury was considered one of the three prime materials of all matter. It was symbolically associated with fluidity and transformation and was represented by the planetary symbol for Mercury (☿).

- **Historic Measurement Tool**: Mercury's high density and liquid state at room temperature made it ideal for use in barometers and thermometers. However, due to its toxicity, it has been largely replaced by safer alternatives in these applications.

- **Cinnabar and Vermilion**: The bright red pigment known as vermilion is derived from the mineral cinnabar, which is a form of mercury sulfide. Historically, it was used in art and decoration, including Chinese lacquerware and Renaissance paintings.

- **Mercury in Folklore**: In folklore and mythology, mercury was often associated with speed and mobility, a characteristic attributed to the Roman god Mercury, known for his swiftness.

- **Dentistry Uses**: Before the health risks were fully understood, mercury was used in dentistry for tooth fillings due to its ability to form amalgams with other metals. Dental amalgams are still used in some places, but their use has decreased significantly.

- **Mercury Vapor Lamps**: Mercury vapor lamps, which emit a bright, bluish light, were once widely used in street lighting. The light is produced by an electric current passing through vaporized mercury.

- **Historical Medicine**: In ancient times, mercury was used in various cultures for supposed health benefits. The ancient Egyptians and Chinese believed that consuming mercury could grant eternal life or heal ailments.

- **Mining and Extraction**: Historically, mercury was obtained by heating cinnabar in a current of air and condensing the vapor. Spain and Italy were historically significant producers of mercury, particularly from the mines of Almadén and Monte Amiata.

- **Role in Gold Mining**: Mercury has been used in gold mining to separate gold from ore. The process involves amalgamating mercury with the gold particles, drawing them out of the ore. This use of mercury has significant environmental and health impacts, particularly in artisanal and small-scale gold mining.

Each of these facts highlights different aspects of mercury's history, uses, and characteristics, painting a picture of a substance that has been both valuable and problematic for human societies.

11. Deadly Delicacies: The Perilous World of Poisonous Mushrooms

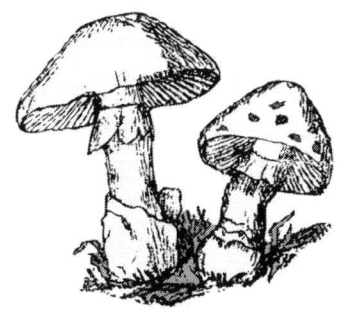

MUSHROOMS

Providing a comprehensive list of all toxic mushroom species worldwide is a monumental task, as there are thousands of mushroom species, and new varieties are still being discovered. However, here is a list of some commonly recognized toxic mushrooms. It's important to note that mushroom identification should always be conducted by experts, as many toxic mushrooms closely resemble edible ones.

1. **Amanita phalloides (Death Cap)**
2. **Amanita virosa (Destroying Angel)**
3. **Amanita muscaria (Fly Agaric)**
4. **Amanita pantherina (Panther Cap)**

5. **Galerina marginata**
6. **Lepiota brunneoincarnata (Deadly Dapperling)**
7. **Lepiota helveola**
8. **Omphalotus olearius (Jack O'Lantern Mushroom)**
9. **Clitocybe dealbata (Ivory Funnel)**
10. **Clitocybe rivulosa (Fool's Funnel)**
11. **Gyromitra esculenta (False Morel)**
12. **Cortinarius rubellus**
13. **Cortinarius orellanus**
14. **Inocybe erubescens**
15. **Entoloma sinuatum**
16. **Paxillus involutus**
17. **Russula emetica (The Sickener)**
18. **Hypholoma fasciculare (Sulphur Tuft)**
19. **Coprinopsis atramentaria (Common Inkcap - toxic in combination with alcohol)**
20. **Coprinus comatus (Shaggy Mane - can become toxic with age)**

Each of these species carries its own risks, from gastrointestinal irritants to potentially fatal toxins like amatoxins. Identification often depends on a range of features, including cap shape and color, gill structure, stem characteristics, spore print color, and habitat.

Please remember, when it comes to wild mushrooms, the rule of thumb is: When in doubt, throw it out.

Misidentification can lead to severe poisoning or even death. Foraging wild mushrooms should only be done with expert knowledge or guidance.

Most Commonly found poisonous mushrooms and their characteristics:

Amanita phalloides (Death Cap)

> **Distinctive Features**: The Death Cap is notorious for its high toxicity. It typically has a greenish or yellowish cap, which can be misleadingly similar in appearance to some edible mushrooms. The cap is usually 5-15 cm in diameter, and the mushroom has a distinctive white, skirt-like ring around the stem.
>
> **Habitat and Distribution**: Common in Europe and now spreading in North America, it's often found in wooded areas, particularly near oak trees.
>
> **Toxic Components**: Contains potent toxins known as amatoxins, which inhibit RNA polymerase II, a crucial enzyme in the synthesis of messenger RNA. This leads to cellular dysfunction and organ failure, particularly in the liver and kidneys.

Amanita muscaria (Fly Agaric)

> **Iconic Appearance**: Known for its bright red cap with white warts, the Fly Agaric is one of the most recognizable mushrooms. The cap color can vary from deep red to orange or yellow.

Psychoactive Properties: It contains psychoactive compounds, including ibotenic acid and muscimol, which can cause a range of effects from mild euphoria and altered perception to delirium and hallucinations.

Cultural Significance: This mushroom has a rich history in various cultures, both as a psychoactive substance and as a symbol in folklore and art. It is believed to have been used by Siberian shamans in religious ceremonies.

Galerina marginata

Deceptive and Deadly: This small, unassuming brown mushroom is extremely poisonous. It resembles edible mushrooms, making it particularly dangerous for foragers.

Habitat: Commonly found on decaying wood, especially in forested areas during the wetter months. It has a bell-shaped or convex cap and a thin stem.

Fatal Toxins: Like the Death Cap, it contains amatoxins, which cause severe liver and kidney damage if ingested.

Lepiota brunneoincarnata (Deadly Dapperling)

Appearance: This mushroom has a smooth, brownish cap, which can appear deceptively similar to some edible varieties. The cap usually measures 4-6 cm in diameter.

Habitat and Distribution: Often found in grassy areas and lawns across Europe and Asia, it prefers calcareous soil.

Toxicity: Contains amatoxins, leading to severe gastrointestinal distress, followed by liver and renal failure if not treated promptly.

How to Identify Poisonous Mushrooms

Identifying poisonous mushrooms is a critical skill, especially for foragers and those interested in wild mushroom harvesting. Misidentification can lead to severe illness or even death. Here's a detailed look at how to distinguish these dangerous fungi.

Beware of Lookalikes: The first and foremost rule in mushroom foraging is understanding that many poisonous mushrooms closely resemble edible varieties. For instance, the deadly Amanita phalloides can look similar to the edible Paddy Straw mushroom. Key identification markers include cap shape, color, gill structure, stem characteristics, and any unique features like rings or veils.

Spore Print Test: One reliable method for mushroom identification is creating a spore print. This involves removing the cap of the mushroom and placing it on a piece of paper or glass. The color of the spores, which will be left on the paper after a few hours, can be a crucial identifier, as different species leave different colored spore prints.

Understanding Habitat: Knowing where certain mushrooms are likely to grow can also aid in identification. Some species prefer wooded areas, while others grow in open fields or near specific types of trees.

Avoiding Risk: For non-experts, the safest approach is to avoid picking wild mushrooms for consumption. Even experienced foragers should cross-reference their finds with multiple reliable guides or consult a mycologist.

Symptoms of Poisoning

Mushroom poisoning symptoms vary depending on the type of mushroom ingested and the amount consumed.

Varying Symptoms: Initial symptoms can include nausea, vomiting, diarrhea, and abdominal pain. Some mushrooms cause more specific symptoms, like the hallucinogenic effects of Amanita muscaria or the intense sweating and salivation caused by Inocybe and Clitocybe species.

Delayed Onset: Particularly dangerous are mushrooms like Amanita phalloides, where symptoms can take 6 to 24 hours to appear, leading to a false sense of security. These symptoms eventually progress to more severe conditions like liver and kidney failure.

Antidotes and Treatment

There are limited options for treating mushroom poisoning, making early medical intervention crucial.

Activated Charcoal and Supportive Care: If ingestion is suspected, activated charcoal may be administered to prevent further absorption of the toxins. Supportive care, including hydration and monitoring of vital functions, is also key.

Liver Transplantation: In cases of severe poisoning, particularly from Amanita species, liver transplantation might be necessary due to irreversible liver damage.

Medicinal Uses

Despite their potential dangers, some mushrooms have beneficial medicinal properties.

Penicillin: The discovery of penicillin from the Penicillium fungus revolutionized medicine, showcasing the potential of fungi in antibiotic development.

Cancer and Immune Research: Certain mushrooms are being researched for their potential in cancer treatment and boosting the immune system. For instance, compounds from mushrooms like Shiitake and Turkey Tail are being studied for their anti-cancer properties.

Famous Poisoning Cases Involving Poisonous Mushrooms

Roman Emperor Claudius: A Political Plot

Ancient Intrigue: Claudius, the Roman Emperor from 41 to 54 AD, is believed to have died after consuming a dish of poisoned mushrooms. While historical accounts vary, many suggest his wife, Agrippina the Younger, orchestrated the poisoning to ensure her son Nero would ascend to the throne.

Historical Debate: The ancient historian Tacitus provides an account of this event, though there is ongoing debate among historians about the veracity and details of this claim. Poisoning, a common practice in Roman political intrigues, was often facilitated by the use of natural toxins like those found in certain mushroom species.

Buddhist Monks in Korea (1994): A Tragic Mistake

Accidental Poisoning: In 1994, a tragic incident occurred in South Korea when a group of Buddhist monks consumed a meal that included wild mushrooms picked from the surrounding area. Unfortunately, the mushrooms were toxic, leading to severe poisoning.

Fatalities and Illness: The incident resulted in several deaths and illnesses among the monks, highlighting the risks associated with foraging and consuming wild mushrooms without proper identification expertise.

Public Awareness: This event raised significant awareness about the dangers of wild mushrooms in South Korea and led to increased public education on mushroom safety.

Additional Noteworthy Cases:

Alexander I of Russia: There is speculation that Alexander I, the Emperor of Russia, may have been poisoned with deadly mushrooms, leading to his mysterious death in 1825. However, like many historical poisoning claims, definitive evidence is lacking.

The Poisoning of Count de Saint-Germain (1774): Count de Saint-Germain, a European adventurer, and alchemist, reportedly died from eating poisonous mushrooms. His death remains shrouded in mystery and is consistent with his enigmatic life.

Conclusion

These cases, ranging from the halls of ancient Rome to a monastery in modern Korea, illustrate the longstanding and sometimes tragic relationship humans have had with poisonous mushrooms. Whether used in political assassinations or mistakenly gathered for nourishment, these fungi have played a significant role in history and continue to be a subject of caution and fascination. Their study not only provides insights into the dangers they pose but also reflects the broader theme of nature's duality as a source of both sustenance and peril.

Interesting Facts:

- **World's Most Poisonous Mushroom**: The Death Cap mushroom (Amanita phalloides) is often considered the most poisonous mushroom in the world. Just one cap is enough to kill a human adult.

- **Bioluminescent Mushrooms**: Some species of poisonous mushrooms are bioluminescent, meaning they can glow in the dark. This phenomenon is thought to attract insects that help spread their spores.

- **Fungi in Warfare**: Historically, there are accounts of poisonous mushrooms being used in warfare. For instance, during the Roman Empire, enemies were known to poison water wells with toxic fungi.

- **Myth and Magic**: In many cultures, poisonous mushrooms were associated with magic and witchcraft. For instance, the Fly Agaric (Amanita muscaria) is often linked to the classic image of witches' brews and fairy tales.

- **Ancient Roman Law Against Poisoning**: The Roman Empire had a specific law, "Lex Cornelia de Sicariis et Veneficiis," against poisoning, including the use of toxic mushrooms, reflecting their awareness of the dangers posed by these fungi.

- **Psychoactive Properties**: Some toxic mushrooms, like the Fly Agaric, have hallucinogenic properties and have been used in various cultural rituals to induce altered states of consciousness.

- **Mushrooms in Literature**: Poisonous mushrooms have a significant presence in literature. They are often used as a plot device in murder mysteries and fantasy stories to add an element of intrigue or danger.

- **Charles Darwin's Interest**: Renowned naturalist Charles Darwin, during his voyage on the HMS Beagle, once unknowingly ate a species of poisonous mushrooms and experienced alarming symptoms, though he recovered.

- **Mushroom Antidotes**: While antidotes for some mushroom toxins exist, such as silibinin for Amanita poisoning, many mushroom poisons lack specific antidotes, making early identification and supportive care crucial.

- **Culinary Delicacy**: In some cultures, mushrooms that are mildly toxic and cause gastrointestinal discomfort are still consumed as delicacies. They are prepared using special cooking methods to reduce their toxicity.

These facts about poisonous mushrooms reveal a world that is not only fraught with danger but also rich in history, culture, and scientific interest, reflecting the intricate and often perilous relationship between humans and the natural world.

12. Polonium: The Radiant Assassin

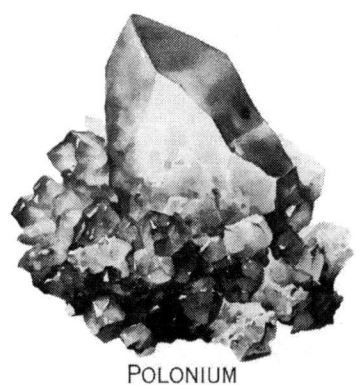

POLONIUM

Historical Background and Properties of Polonium

Discovery and Naming

Marie Curie's Landmark Discovery: Polonium was discovered by Marie Curie and her husband Pierre in 1898 during their research on radioactivity. They extracted it from pitchblende, a mineral rich in uranium, after noticing that the ore was more radioactive than uranium itself should be.

Tribute to Poland: Marie Curie named the element "polonium" in honor of her native country, Poland, which was then under political partition and oppression. This act of naming was also a bold statement of national pride and political defiance.

Early Challenges: Isolating polonium was challenging due to its extreme rarity. The Curies' process of refining pitchblende to extract polonium was laborious and involved processing tons of the ore to obtain a tiny amount of the element.

Physical Characteristics and Isotopes

Appearance and Structure: Polonium is a silvery-gray metalloid that resembles its periodic table neighbors, bismuth and tellurium, in physical appearance and chemical behavior. At room temperature, it exists in a solid state.

Radioactive Nature: Polonium is highly radioactive and emits alpha particles. It has 33 known isotopes, all of which are radioactive. Polonium-210, the most famous isotope due to its use in the Litvinenko case, has a half-life of 138 days.

Decay and Radiation: The alpha radiation emitted by polonium is not penetrating and can be stopped by a sheet of paper or even the skin. However, if ingested or inhaled, polonium-210 is extremely lethal due to its ability to cause significant biological damage internally.

Source, Rarity, and Collection

Rare Occurrence: Polonium is extremely rare in nature. It is found in uranium ores but only in minute quantities, approximately 100 micrograms of polonium for every ton of uranium ore.

Extraction and Synthesis: Polonium is typically produced artificially in nuclear reactors or particle accelerators. This production is necessary for most practical applications due to its scarcity in nature and the impracticality of extracting it from uranium ore.

Industrial and Scientific Uses

Heat Generation: Due to its ability to generate heat through radioactive decay, polonium has been used in thermoelectric devices, such as those in space probes where solar power is ineffective.

Static Elimination: Another application of polonium is in devices designed to eliminate static electricity in industrial settings, particularly in machinery where static could pose a hazard or interfere with electronic components.

Scientific Research: Polonium's intense radioactivity makes it useful in certain areas of scientific research, including physics and chemistry, although its use is strictly controlled due to the associated health risks.

Polonium's discovery marked a significant milestone in the field of radiochemistry and opened up new avenues in scientific research. However, its high radioactivity and toxicity require careful handling and strict regulations to prevent its misuse or accidental exposure.

The Infamous Litvinenko Case

The Poisoning

A Stealthy Attack: On November 1, 2006, Alexander Litvinenko, a former Russian spy and fierce critic of the Kremlin, fell ill after meeting with two Russian men at a London hotel. What appeared initially to be a case of food poisoning quickly escalated into a matter of international intrigue when it was revealed he had been poisoned with a rare and highly lethal substance: polonium-210.

Symptoms and Diagnosis: Litvinenko's condition deteriorated rapidly, with hair loss and a severe decline in his immune system. Doctors were baffled until they discovered the cause of his illness was radioactive polonium-210, a discovery that turned a medical mystery into a political scandal.

Investigation and Aftermath

Tracing the Poison: The investigation into Litvinenko's death was extensive and complex. Investigators found traces of polonium-210 in various locations across London, including the hotel where he had met with the Russian individuals, a sushi restaurant, and even on airplanes that had traveled between London and Moscow.

Culprits and Motives: The British inquiry pointed to Andrei Lugovoi and Dmitry Kovtun, the men who met with Litvinenko, as the primary suspects. The investigation concluded that the murder was likely a state-sponsored assassination, sanctioned at the highest levels of the Russian government, possibly as retribution for Litvinenko's public criticism of President Vladimir Putin.

International Fallout: The case severely strained diplomatic relations between the United Kingdom and Russia. It raised serious concerns about state-sponsored terrorism and the use of radioactive materials in assassinations, leading to calls for tighter regulation and security measures globally.

Impact on International Relations

Diplomatic Tensions: The incident led to a significant deterioration in UK-Russia relations. The UK expelled Russian diplomats, and Russia responded in kind. The mutual distrust and worsening relations marked a significant low point in the post-Cold War era.

Security Concerns: The use of polonium-210, a highly controlled radioactive substance, in a public assassination raised alarms about nuclear security and the illicit trafficking of radioactive materials.

Legacy: The Litvinenko case remains a symbol of the dark art of political assassination in the 21st century. It not only highlighted the risks associated with radiological substances but also showed how these materials could be used in geopolitical power plays.

The Litvinenko case stands out as a stark reminder of the lethal capabilities of radioactive substances when misused and the lengths to which some regimes may go to silence dissent. It underscores the importance of international cooperation and vigilance in preventing the misuse of nuclear and radiological materials.

The Deadly Science of Radioactive Decay: Understanding Polonium's Lethality

Radioactive Properties of Polonium-210

Alpha Particle Emission: Polonium-210 decays by emitting alpha particles, which are helium-4 nuclei consisting of two protons and two neutrons. These particles are heavily charged and highly energetic.

Penetration and Range: Despite their high energy, alpha particles have a very short range and cannot penetrate deeply into materials; even a piece of paper or human skin can stop them. However, their high ionization power makes them extremely dangerous when they come into direct contact with living tissues, such as when inhaled or ingested.

Radiation Exposure and Contamination: Polonium-210 can contaminate air, water, and food. Once inside the body, it irradiates internal organs, particularly affecting rapidly dividing cells like those in the bone marrow and the gastrointestinal tract.

Mechanism of Toxicity

Cellular Damage: When polonium decays inside the body, its alpha emissions bombard cells at a close range, causing intense ionization effects. This leads to severe DNA damage, disrupting cellular function and causing cell death.

Acute Radiation Syndrome (ARS): High doses of alpha radiation from polonium can result in ARS, characterized by nausea, vomiting, hair loss, and damage to the bone marrow and the gastrointestinal tract. In severe cases, ARS can lead to organ failure and death within days or weeks.

Long-term Effects: Survivors of initial polonium exposure may suffer long-term effects, including an increased risk of developing cancer, due to the genetic damage caused by the radiation.

Invisible and Silent Killer

Undetectable by Ordinary Means: Polonium's danger is compounded by its difficulty to detect. It does not emit gamma rays, which are typically used to detect radioactivity, and its alpha particles are easily shielded.

Stealthy Nature: This characteristic makes polonium a stealthy poison, as it leaves no sensory clues like taste or smell. Its symptoms can mimic those of other illnesses, making diagnosis challenging without specific tests.

Lack of Antidote and Treatment Challenges

No Effective Antidote: There is no antidote for polonium-210 poisoning. Once it has entered the body, the focus of treatment is on supportive care and limiting further exposure.

Treatment Strategies: Treatment may involve chelation therapy, which can help remove some heavy metals from the body, but its effectiveness against polonium is limited. Supportive treatments also include managing symptoms, providing fluids, and treating infections.

The deadly science of polonium's radioactive decay lies in its ability to cause severe internal damage while remaining undetectable until symptoms arise. Its role in high-profile poisoning cases underscores the need for caution in handling radioactive materials and the importance of nuclear security in preventing illicit use.

Intriguing Facts About Polonium:

- **Nobel Prize Connections**: Polonium was a key element in the research that led to Marie Curie receiving the Nobel Prize. She won the Nobel Prize in Physics in 1903 (shared with her husband Pierre Curie and Henri Becquerel) and again in Chemistry in 1911, making her the first person to win Nobel Prizes in two different sciences.

- **First Self-Luminous Paint**: Polonium was used in the early 20th century to create the first self-luminous paints. These paints were used on watch and clock faces because polonium's alpha radiation caused certain materials to glow.

- **Spacecraft Heat Source**: Due to its ability to release heat upon decaying, polonium has been used as a heat source in lunar and planetary rovers, including the Lunokhod rovers deployed by the Soviet Union.

- **Atomic Number and Symbol**: Polonium has the atomic number 84 and is represented by the symbol 'Po' on the periodic table.

- **Extremely Rare in Nature**: Polonium is so rare that it's estimated to be about 100 billion times less abundant than uranium in the Earth's crust.

- **A Curie Family Affair**: Polonium's discovery was a family affair. Marie Curie's husband, Pierre, and her physicist brother-in-law, Jacques Curie, played significant roles in researching and identifying the element.

- **Highly Unstable**: All isotopes of polonium are radioactive, and the element has no stable isotopes. Its most stable isotope, polonium-209, has a half-life of 125.2 years.

- **Short-Lived Isotopes**: Some isotopes of polonium have very short half-lives. For instance, polonium-212 has a half-life of just 0.3 microseconds.

- **Industrial Thickness Gauging**: Polonium-210 has been used in devices to measure the thickness of paper, sheet metal, and other materials due to its ability to emit alpha particles that can penetrate small distances.

- **Health Hazards in Production**: Workers involved in the extraction and processing of polonium must follow stringent safety protocols due to its intense radioactivity and the risk of radiation poisoning.

13. Ricin: Nature's Lethal Protein

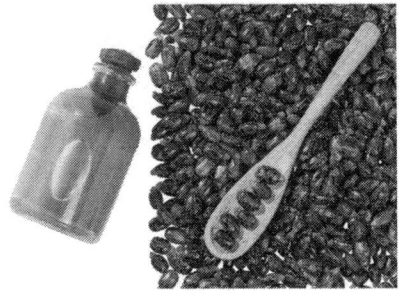

CASTER OIL BEANS / RICIN

Sources and Historical Context

Derived from Castor Beans

Extraction Process: Ricin is extracted from the waste mash produced during the processing of castor beans for castor oil. Although the oil itself is safe and widely used, the leftover mash contains high concentrations of this deadly toxin.

Geographical Spread: The castor oil plant is native to the southeastern Mediterranean Basin, Eastern Africa, and India, but it has been introduced to other regions, including the Americas and Europe. It thrives in both tropical and temperate climates.

Ancient Use and Recognition

Historical Awareness: While ancient civilizations, including the Egyptians, used castor oil for various purposes, there is evidence to suggest they were aware of the bean's toxic nature. Historical records indicate caution was advised when handling and processing the beans.

Cultural Significance: In various cultures, the castor oil plant has been surrounded by myths and legends, often related to its dual nature of healing and harm. Its seeds were sometimes used in traditional rituals and medicinal practices, albeit with extreme caution.

World War I and Beyond

Military Research: During World War I, the American, British, and Canadian armies experimented with ricin as a potential chemical warfare agent. The idea was to use ricin in artillery shells to incapacitate enemy troops.

Cold War Developments: Research into ricin as a biological weapon continued during the Cold War, with studies focusing on its stability, dispersion methods, and potential as an incapacitating agent.

International Control: Despite these studies, ricin has been relatively less utilized as a weapon compared to other chemical agents. Its production and use are controlled under the Chemical Weapons Convention.

Castor Bean Popularity

Agricultural and Industrial Use: The castor bean plant is widely cultivated for its oil, used in lubricants, paints, varnishes, and other industrial products. The oil is also used medicinally as a laxative and in skin care products.

Ornamental Plant: The plant is also popular in gardens and landscapes for its striking appearance, characterized by large, star-shaped leaves that can be green or reddish-purple. However, gardeners are cautioned about the potential risks, especially in households with children and pets.

Resilience and Spread: The plant is known for its hardiness and ability to grow in poor soil, making it a resilient species. In some areas, it has become an invasive species, spreading beyond cultivated fields.

Famous Incidents Involving Ricin:

Georgi Markov Assassination (1978)

Cold War Espionage: The assassination of Georgi Markov, a Bulgarian dissident and journalist, in 1978, remains one of the most infamous uses of ricin as a tool for political assassination. On September 7, while waiting for a bus on London's Waterloo Bridge, Markov was jabbed in the leg with an umbrella, which was modified to inject a tiny pellet containing ricin.

Delayed Fatality: Markov felt a sharp pain at the site of the jab but initially thought little of it. However, he developed a high fever and died four days later. An autopsy revealed the presence of a ricin-laced pellet in his leg.

International Mystery: This high-profile case turned into a major international incident, with suspicions pointing towards the Bulgarian secret service and the KGB.

Ricin Letters in the United States

Targeting Officials: In the early 2000s, the United States saw a series of incidents where ricin was sent through the mail, targeting politicians and public figures. These cases did not result in fatalities but caused alarm due to the potential for harm.

Increased Security Measures: These incidents led to heightened security measures, especially in handling mail for government officials, and raised public awareness about the potential use of biological agents in terroristic threats.

Terrorism Attempts

Planned Attacks: Ricin has been discovered in connection with various terrorist plots. Due to its high toxicity and relative ease of production, it has been considered by extremist groups for use in attacks.

Preventive Measures: Law enforcement agencies worldwide have become more vigilant in monitoring for ricin production and possession, often intercepting plots before they come to fruition.

Other Notable Cases

Roger Von Bergendorff Poisoning (2008): In Las Vegas, Roger Von Bergendorff poisoned himself accidentally with ricin, which he had produced in his hotel room. This incident caused a major public health scare.

Shannon Richardson Mailing (2013): Actress Shannon Richardson was arrested for sending ricin-laced letters to President Barack Obama and New York City Mayor Michael Bloomberg. She was sentenced to 18 years in prison.

Alleged North Korean Use: There have been allegations of North Korea using ricin in assassination plots, though these claims are surrounded by secrecy and lack public evidence.

Ricin's history in assassinations, terror plots, and accidental poisonings illustrates its potency and the risks associated with this naturally occurring toxin. These incidents have contributed to the development of stricter regulations and awareness about the dangers of biological agents.

Interesting Facts:

- **Extremely Small Lethal Dose**: Ricin is so potent that a dose as small as a few grains of table salt can be lethal to an adult if inhaled, injected, or ingested.

- **No Taste or Smell**: Ricin is particularly dangerous because it is colorless, odorless, and tasteless, making it difficult to detect when added to food or water.

- **Rapid Breakdown**: Ricin degrades quickly in nature. In water, for example, ricin can break down within days to a week, which makes it less likely to cause long-term contamination.

- **Ancient Weaponry**: Historical records suggest that ricin has been known and possibly used as a poison for centuries. Some ancient texts hint at the use of ricin-laced food and drinks in political assassinations.

- **Use in Cancer Research**: Despite its toxicity, researchers have investigated using modified ricin to attack and kill cancer cells. The idea is to link ricin to antibodies that specifically target cancer cells, minimizing the toxin's effect on healthy cells.

- **Castor Bean Plant and Wildlife**: Interestingly, while the castor bean plant's seeds are toxic to humans and many animals, some wildlife species have developed a tolerance or resistance to ricin, allowing them to consume the seeds without harm.

- **Ricin in Literature and Media**: Ricin has been featured in several novels, TV shows, and movies, often as a plot device in murder mysteries and espionage stories. Its infamous reputation has made it a symbol of covert operations and intrigue.

- **Symptom Onset**: The onset of symptoms from ricin poisoning can vary from a couple of hours to a day, depending on the route of exposure and the dose received.

- **Biological Warfare Regulations**: Due to its potential as a bioterrorism agent, the production and possession of ricin are highly regulated under the Biological Weapons Convention.

- **Diagnostic Challenges**: Diagnosing ricin poisoning can be challenging, as its symptoms can resemble those of other illnesses, and there's no widely available, specific test for ricin exposure.

14. Strychnine: Convulsions and Crime

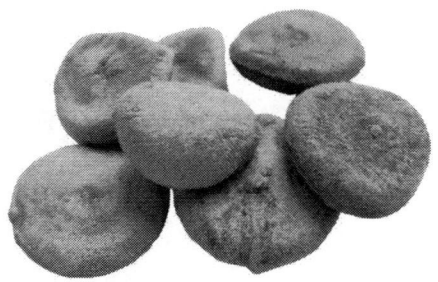

NUX VOMICA - STRYCHNINE

Origins and Extraction:

Derived from Nux Vomica Tree

> **Botanical Background**: The Nux Vomica tree, from which strychnine is derived, is a medium-sized tree with a short trunk and a dense crown. It bears small, greenish-white flowers and orange-colored berries. The tree is commonly found in coastal and wetland areas of India and Southeast Asia.
>
> **Toxic Seeds**: The seeds of the Nux Vomica tree, about the size of a large button, are the primary source of strychnine. These seeds are notably hard and dense, with a disc-like shape and a slightly pitted surface.

Cultural Significance: In some Asian cultures, the Nux Vomica tree has been surrounded by superstitions and fears due to its highly toxic nature. It's often associated with various local legends and folklore.

Extraction Process

Initial Processing: To extract strychnine, the seeds of the Nux Vomica tree are first dried and then crushed into a fine powder. This powder contains several alkaloids, including strychnine and brucine.

Solvent Extraction: The powdered seeds are treated with alcohol, typically ethanol, which dissolves the alkaloids. This process may be repeated several times to increase the yield.

Refinement: The alcoholic solution is then evaporated to concentrate the alkaloids. Further chemical processing, involving acid-base extraction and crystallization techniques, isolates pure strychnine.

Historical Use:

Pesticide and Rodenticide: Due to its potent toxicity, strychnine was historically used as a pesticide, especially for controlling rodents in agriculture and urban settings. Its use in this manner has significantly declined due to the risks to wildlife and humans, as well as the availability of safer alternatives.

Performance Enhancer: In the late 19th and early 20th centuries, strychnine was occasionally used as a stimulant and performance enhancer by athletes. This practice was dangerous and often led to adverse effects or fatalities.

Medicinal Applications:

Traditional Medicine: In Ayurveda and traditional Chinese medicine, strychnine, in extremely small doses, was used for its stimulant properties. It was believed to invigorate the body, treat digestive issues, and even act as an aphrodisiac.

Controversial Usage: The medical use of strychnine has always been controversial due to its narrow therapeutic index. While it was included in some pharmacopeias in the past, its use in modern medicine is virtually nonexistent due to the availability of safer and more effective drugs.

The story of strychnine is a compelling example of how substances derived from nature can have both beneficial and harmful aspects. Its historical use, both as a poison and a medicine, reflects the complex relationship between natural compounds and their applications in human society.

Notable Cases in Literature and Reality Involving Strychnine:

Literary Appearances

Sherlock Holmes and the Classic Mystery: In "The Adventure of the Speckled Band," one of Sir Arthur Conan Doyle's most famous Sherlock Holmes stories, strychnine is used as a pivotal element of the plot, showcasing Doyle's knowledge of contemporary forensic science.

Agatha Christie's Use of Strychnine: Renowned mystery writer Agatha Christie, who had a professional background in pharmacy, frequently used strychnine in her novels, including "The Mysterious Affair at Styles," where the poison plays a central role in the murder mystery.

Symbol of Sinister Intrigue: Strychnine's presence in literature often symbolizes the sinister and dark aspects of human nature, making it a favorite choice for stories involving murder and deception.

Famous Poisoning Cases:

The Charles Bravo Case (1876): The death of British attorney Charles Bravo, which resulted from acute strychnine poisoning, led to a sensational and highly publicized inquest. Despite extensive investigations, the case remained unsolved, becoming one of the most infamous unsolved poisoning cases in British history.

Dr. Thomas Neill Cream: In the late 19th century, Dr. Thomas Neill Cream was a notorious serial killer who used strychnine as his murder weapon. He was eventually caught and executed, his crimes contributing to the fearsome reputation of strychnine.

Criminal Use:

Rat Poison Turned Murder Weapon: Due to its historical use as a rat poison, strychnine has been accessible and thus employed in numerous criminal poisonings. However, its strong, bitter taste and the painful symptoms it causes have often led to early detection, sometimes thwarting criminal intentions.

Notorious Assassinations:

Alleged Political Uses: While concrete evidence is often lacking, there have been various allegations and suspicions regarding the use of strychnine in political assassinations. These claims are part of the broader narrative of poisons being used as covert tools in political power struggles.

The Mystery of Alexander Perepilichnyy (2012): Russian businessman Alexander Perepilichnyy, who died in the UK under mysterious circumstances, was speculated to have been poisoned with strychnine, though the inquest yielded an open verdict.

The role of strychnine in both fiction and reality has often intersected, with its dramatic and unmistakable symptoms making it a substance of intrigue and horror. Its use in literature reflects a deep cultural understanding of its potency and danger, while real-life cases underscore the grim reality of this potent poison. Whether in the pages of a novel or the dark annals of criminal history, strychnine remains a symbol of lethal cunning and a testament to the darker aspects of human ingenuity.

How Strychnine Wreaks Havoc on the Nervous System:

Mechanism of Action

Interference with Neurotransmitters: Strychnine's primary mechanism of action is its interference with the neurotransmitter glycine, which normally acts as an inhibitory neurotransmitter in the spinal cord and brainstem. Glycine plays a crucial role in dampening neuronal activity and preventing muscle spasms.

Disruption of Neural Control: By blocking the inhibitory action of glycine, strychnine disrupts the normal balance of neural signals. This leads to an overstimulation of neurons, causing excessive muscle contractions and heightened reflex responses.

Rapid Onset of Symptoms: The effects of strychnine poisoning manifest quickly, often within minutes of ingestion, due to its rapid absorption and distribution in the central nervous system.

Symptoms of Poisoning:

Muscle Spasms and Stiffness: The initial symptoms include muscle stiffness, particularly in the face and neck, followed by painful muscle spasms. These spasms can be triggered by minimal stimuli, such as a slight touch or noise.

Violent Convulsions: As the poisoning progresses, the victim experiences violent and painful convulsions. These can be so intense that they lead to muscle tears, fractures, and joint dislocations.

Characteristic "Risus Sardonicus": A hallmark of strychnine poisoning is the appearance of a sustained spasm of the facial muscles that resembles a grimace, known as "risus sardonicus".

Respiratory Failure and Death:

Asphyxiation: The most common cause of death from strychnine poisoning is asphyxiation. The convulsions can impair breathing by causing a sustained contraction of the respiratory muscles, making it impossible for the victim to breathe.

Exhaustion of the Respiratory System: Even if the initial convulsions are survived, the continuous muscle activity can lead to exhaustion and collapse of the respiratory system.

No Known Antidote and Treatment Approaches:

Lack of Specific Antidote: Currently, there is no specific antidote for strychnine poisoning.

Treatment focuses on managing symptoms and preventing complications.

Symptom Management: This includes administering muscle relaxants, sedatives, and anticonvulsants to control convulsions. Mechanical ventilation may be necessary to support breathing.

Supportive Care: Treatment also involves supportive care, including hydration and monitoring of kidney function, as the body works to metabolize and eliminate the toxin.

In summary, strychnine's potent action on the nervous system makes it one of the most dangerous poisons. Its ability to cause severe and often fatal convulsions has made it a substance of both historical and contemporary concern in the field of toxicology.

Interesting Facts:

- **Early Medical Use**: Despite its toxicity, strychnine was once used in conventional medicine, especially in the 19th and early 20th centuries. It was prescribed in small doses as a treatment for a wide variety of ailments, including depression, migraines, and other neurological disorders.

- **Natural Pest Deterrent**: Certain animals have developed an evolutionary aversion to the smell and taste of strychnine, effectively using it as a natural defense mechanism against predation.

- **Detection in Forensic Science**: Strychnine has a unique place in the history of forensic science. It was one of the first poisons to be identified in a forensic investigation, leading to advancements in toxicology as a science.

- **Use in Performance Enhancement**: In the late 19th and early 20th centuries, strychnine was occasionally used by athletes as a performance-enhancing drug due to its stimulant properties, before the advent of modern doping regulations.

- **Bitter Taste**: Strychnine is known for its extremely bitter taste, which can be detected in very dilute solutions. This property has occasionally led to its detection in attempted poisonings.

- **Role in Literature**: Beyond detective stories, strychnine has appeared in various literary works, symbolizing treachery and hidden dangers. It's often used to heighten drama or as a plot device in murder mysteries.

- **Symbolism in Art**: In art and literature, strychnine has been used symbolically to represent bitterness, both literally and metaphorically, in human relationships and experiences.

- **Strychnine in the Animal Kingdom**: Some species of birds and other wildlife have been known to eat Nux Vomica seeds without apparent harm, suggesting a natural resistance or tolerance to strychnine.

- **Environmental Persistence**: Strychnine is not very persistent in the environment and tends to break down relatively quickly, which has limited its long-term environmental impact.

- **Regulation and Control**: Due to its high toxicity, the sale and distribution of strychnine are heavily regulated in many countries, and its use is subject to strict legal controls to prevent misuse and accidental poisonings.

These facts illustrate the complex history of strychnine, highlighting its transformation from a widely used substance in medicine and athletics to a recognized and regulated poison.

15. Other Notable Poisons and Their Associated Murders or Assassination Attempts

Thallium: The Silent Assassin

Chemical Profile: Thallium is a heavy, soft, gray metal that, when purified, is both tasteless and odorless. It can be highly toxic even in small amounts and is particularly insidious because symptoms of poisoning often mimic those of other illnesses.

Graham Frederick Young: Known as the "Teacup Poisoner," Young was infamous for his use of thallium in the 1960s and 1970s in the UK. He was fascinated by chemistry and poisons from a young age and began experimenting with them on family members, classmates, and later, co-workers. His precise dosing and knowledge of the chemical made him a particularly chilling figure.

Symptoms and Detection: Thallium poisoning symptoms include hair loss, nerve damage, and eventual organ failure. Because of its slow-acting nature, victims often suffered for weeks or months before the cause was identified.

Historical Use: Before its toxicity was fully understood, thallium was used in rat poisons and insecticides. Its unrestricted availability during the early and mid-20th century made it a choice weapon for several murderers.

Restrictions and Regulations: The rise in thallium poisoning cases, both accidental and intentional, led to stricter regulations and a decline in its availability for the general public.

Dimethylmercury: A Silent and Deadly Chemical

The Tragic Case of Karen Wetterhahn

A Tragic Accident: Karen Wetterhahn, a respected professor of chemistry at Dartmouth College, experienced a fatal encounter with dimethylmercury in 1996. This incident highlights the extreme danger posed by certain chemical compounds, even in seemingly minimal amounts.

The Incident: Wetterhahn was conducting research on heavy metal toxicity and was using dimethylmercury as a standard for nuclear magnetic resonance (NMR) spectroscopy. Despite following standard safety protocols and wearing latex gloves, a few drops of the compound penetrated her glove and came into contact with her skin.

Delayed Symptoms and Diagnosis: The symptoms of mercury poisoning didn't manifest immediately. It was only months later that Wetterhahn began experiencing the first signs of mercury poisoning, which quickly progressed to full-blown toxic encephalopathy, a severe brain damage.

Fatal Outcome: Despite aggressive chelation therapy, the damage was irreversible. Wetterhahn passed away less than a year after the initial exposure, underscoring the insidious nature of dimethylmercury.

Properties and Dangers of Dimethylmercury

Chemical Characteristics: Dimethylmercury is a colorless, volatile liquid at room temperature. It's one of the strongest known neurotoxins and is absorbed through the skin rapidly and easily.

Uses and Handling: The compound is used in certain scientific applications, particularly in spectroscopy and as a reference standard in some laboratory procedures. Following Wetterhahn's death, safety protocols for handling dimethylmercury were significantly revised.

Toxicity and Protection: Dimethylmercury's ability to penetrate standard laboratory safety gloves quickly made it particularly dangerous. Researchers now use highly specialized gloves and take extra precautions when handling this compound.

Mechanism of Toxicity: As an organomercury compound, dimethylmercury is highly lipid-soluble, allowing it to easily pass through the blood-brain barrier and accumulate in the brain. It disrupts the central nervous system and can lead to severe neurological damage.

Impact on Safety Standards

Reevaluation of Laboratory Safety: The tragedy of Karen Wetterhahn led to a reevaluation of safety protocols in laboratories worldwide. It highlighted the need for more stringent safety measures and better education about the risks of working with highly toxic substances.

Legacy in Chemical Safety: Wetterhahn's death serves as a somber reminder of the risks associated with chemical research and the utmost importance of safety in the handling of toxic substances.

Dioxin: A Political Poison

The Poisoning of Viktor Yushchenko

Incident Overview: In September 2004, during a heated presidential campaign in Ukraine, Viktor Yushchenko, then a candidate, fell victim to a high-profile poisoning incident. Yushchenko's illness was initially mysterious, characterized by severe abdominal pain and facial disfigurement.

Diagnosis and Effects: It was later determined that Yushchenko had been poisoned with dioxin, a highly toxic and environmentally persistent compound. The poisoning caused chloracne, a severe skin condition, and disfigured Yushchenko's face with cysts, pustules, and lesions.

Survival and Long-term Health Impact: Yushchenko survived the assassination attempt but suffered chronic health issues as a result of the dioxin poisoning. The long-term health implications included facial disfigurement, weakness, and potentially compromised organ functions.

Properties and Risks of Dioxin

Chemical Characteristics: Dioxins are a group of chemically-related compounds that are environmental pollutants. They are byproducts of various industrial processes and are known for their persistence in the environment and in the human body.

Toxicity: Dioxins are highly toxic and can cause reproductive and developmental problems, damage the immune system, interfere with hormones, and also cause cancer.

Mode of Poisoning: Dioxin poisoning typically occurs through ingestion of contaminated food. In Yushchenko's case, the high concentration and the symptoms suggested a deliberate poisoning rather than accidental exposure.

Political Ramifications of Yushchenko's Poisoning

Impact on Ukrainian Politics: The incident played a significant role in the narrative of the 2004 Ukrainian presidential election. Yushchenko's survival and continued candidacy garnered him considerable public sympathy and support.

International Relations: The poisoning of a prominent political figure in such a manner led to international outrage and speculation about the involvement of political opponents. It strained Ukraine's relations with neighboring countries, particularly Russia.

Legacy in Public Health and Safety: The Yushchenko incident highlighted the dangers posed by toxic compounds such as dioxin and raised concerns about the security of high-profile individuals. It also brought attention to the need for stricter controls and better detection of environmental toxins.

VX Nerve Agent: A Lethal Tool in Covert Operations

Assassination of Kim Jong-nam

High-Profile Incident: On February 13, 2017, Kim Jong-nam, the half-brother of North Korean leader Kim Jong-un, was assassinated at Kuala Lumpur International Airport in a shocking and brazen attack that drew global attention.

Method of Assassination: Kim Jong-nam was attacked by two women who smeared a substance on his face, later identified as VX nerve agent. The use of this highly potent toxin in a crowded public area was particularly alarming.

Immediate Effects and Death: Kim Jong-nam exhibited symptoms almost immediately and sought medical help at the airport. Despite rapid response, he died within hours of the attack, underscoring the extreme potency of the VX agent.

Suspected State-Sponsored Assassination: The use of VX, a substance classified as a weapon of mass destruction, led to widespread speculation about state-sponsored involvement. Given the complexity of handling and deploying VX, experts suggested that the assassination was likely orchestrated at a high level.

Properties and Risks of VX Nerve Agent

Chemical Characteristics: VX is a synthetic compound and is classified as a nerve agent, one of the most toxic and fast-acting substances known in chemical warfare.

Mechanism of Action: VX operates by inhibiting an enzyme called acetylcholinesterase, leading to an accumulation of acetylcholine in the nerve synapses. This causes continuous stimulation of the muscles, glands, and central nervous system.

Symptoms of Exposure: Exposure to VX can cause convulsions, paralysis, respiratory failure, and death. Even a tiny droplet absorbed through the skin can be fatal within minutes to hours.

Difficulty in Detection and Treatment: VX is odorless and tasteless, making it difficult to detect. Immediate treatment is crucial for survival, including administration of antidotes such as atropine and pralidoxime.

International Implications of the VX Assassination

Violation of Chemical Weapons Convention: The use of VX nerve agent in the assassination was a clear violation of the Chemical Weapons Convention, raising serious international legal and security concerns.

Diplomatic Fallout: The incident strained Malaysia's diplomatic relations with North Korea and led to a reevaluation of security measures in international airports and other public spaces.

Focus on Chemical Weapons Proliferation: The assassination brought renewed attention to the issue of chemical weapons proliferation and the need for rigorous international monitoring and control.

Hydrogen Cyanide: A Chemical With a Dark History

The Jonestown Massacre: A Tragic Use of Hydrogen Cyanide

Mass Suicide and Murder: In November 1978, one of the most harrowing events involving hydrogen cyanide occurred at the Jonestown commune in Guyana. Led by cult leader Jim Jones, over 900 members of the Peoples Temple agricultural commune died in a mass suicide-murder. The majority of the victims were poisoned with a cyanide-laced drink, infamously referred to as "Kool-Aid," although it was actually a different brand of flavored drink mix.

Mechanics of the Poisoning: The cyanide used at Jonestown was reportedly stolen from a local jeweler and mixed into large containers of the flavored drink. Many of the victims, including numerous children, were forced to ingest the poison, while others willingly participated in what was termed a "revolutionary act" by Jones.

Aftermath and Impact: The Jonestown massacre stands as one of the largest mass deaths in a single event and left a permanent mark on popular culture and the collective psyche. It raised global awareness about the dangers of cults and the potential for manipulation under charismatic leadership.

Properties and Risks of Hydrogen Cyanide

Chemical Profile: Hydrogen cyanide (HCN) is a highly poisonous compound that interferes with the body's ability to use oxygen. It can be released from certain industrial processes and is present in cigarette smoke.

Rapid Action: Hydrogen cyanide acts quickly, making it a particularly dangerous poison. Inhalation or ingestion of even small amounts can lead to rapid respiratory failure and death.

Historical Use: Aside from Jonestown, hydrogen cyanide has been used historically as a fumigant, in chemical warfare, and in the gas chambers of the Holocaust during World War II.

Symptoms of Poisoning: Symptoms of cyanide poisoning include headache, dizziness, confusion, shortness of breath, and loss of consciousness. In high enough doses, it can cause death within minutes.

Broader Implications of the Jonestown Massacre

Cult Dynamics and Psychological Control: The Jonestown event remains a significant case study in psychology, sociology, and religious studies, illustrating the extreme potential for manipulation and control within cults.

Emergency Response and Forensic Investigations: The response to the Jonestown tragedy highlighted the need for international cooperation in emergency situations and the challenges faced in forensic investigations of mass casualty events.

Legacy and Cultural References: The phrase "drinking the Kool-Aid," although derived inaccurately from the Jonestown massacre, has become a colloquialism in popular culture, referring to blind conformity or unquestioning loyalty.

Morphine/Heroin: A Tool for a Serial Killer in Medicine

The Case of Dr. Harold Shipman

Deadly Practice: Dr. Harold Shipman, dubbed "Dr. Death," was a respected general practitioner in the UK who was convicted in 2000 of the murder of 15 of his patients, though later investigations suggested he may have been responsible for the deaths of up to 250 patients over a 23-year period.

Method of Murder: Shipman's modus operandi involved administering lethal overdoses of diamorphine (the medical name for pharmaceutical heroin) to his patients. He targeted the elderly and vulnerable, often forging medical records to cover his tracks.

Discovery and Investigation: Shipman's crimes were eventually uncovered after a local undertaker noticed an unusually high number of cremation certificates for Shipman's patients. A subsequent investigation revealed a pattern of administering lethal doses of diamorphine, falsifying medical records, and then signing death certificates attributing the deaths to natural causes.

Impact and Aftermath: The Shipman case is one of the most shocking and extensive cases of serial murder in modern history. It led to significant changes in medical practice and legal procedures in the UK, including changes to the regulation of controlled substances and reforms in the death certification process.

Morphine and Heroin in Medical Context

Pharmaceutical Use: Morphine, derived from the opium poppy, is a powerful painkiller used in medicine for severe pain. Diamorphine (heroin) is a semi-synthetic opioid, which, in a medical context, is used for its effective pain-relieving properties, particularly in end-of-life care.

Risks and Controls: Both morphine and diamorphine can be highly addictive and have a high potential for abuse. Their medical use is strictly regulated, and they are classified as controlled substances in many countries.

Overdose Effects: An overdose of these opioids can lead to respiratory depression, a decrease in heart rate, unconsciousness, and death. The fine line between a therapeutic dose and a lethal dose makes these substances particularly dangerous if misused.

Broader Implications of the Shipman Case

Trust in Medical Professionals: The Shipman case severely impacted public trust in general practitioners and the medical profession. It raised questions about the ease with which a trusted doctor could exploit his position to commit murder.

Regulatory Changes: The case led to a reexamination of prescription practices and the monitoring of controlled substances in the UK. It also prompted the development of stricter guidelines for death certification and investigation.

Cultural and Psychological Impact: The case has been the subject of numerous documentaries, books, and studies, contributing to the discourse on medical ethics, the psychology of serial killers, and the safeguarding of vulnerable patients.

Nicotine: A Toxic Agent Beyond Addiction

Nicotine as a Murder Weapon

The 2014 German Case: In a rare instance of nicotine being used as a poison for murder, a German woman was convicted in 2014 for killing her boyfriend. She administered a lethal dose of nicotine to him through an injection, leading to his death. This case is one of the few modern instances where nicotine was deliberately used to commit murder.

Method of Administration: The use of an injection in this case is notable because it allowed for a concentrated dose of nicotine to be delivered directly into the bloodstream, resulting in rapid and potent toxic effects.

Properties and Risks of Nicotine

Chemical Profile: Nicotine is a naturally occurring alkaloid found in tobacco plants. It acts as a natural insecticide for the plant. In humans, it stimulates the nervous system, which is why it is both addictive and potentially toxic in high doses.

Symptoms of Nicotine Poisoning: The symptoms of nicotine poisoning, also known as nicotine overdose, can include nausea, vomiting, increased heart rate, high blood pressure, seizures, and, in extreme cases, respiratory failure and death.

Recognizability: One of the reasons nicotine is less commonly used as a poison in murders is its recognizable symptoms, which are similar to those of tobacco overdose. Additionally, the widespread awareness of nicotine due to its presence in tobacco products makes it a less desirable choice for covert poisoning.

Nicotine in Forensic Investigations

Detection and Analysis: Modern forensic toxicology can detect nicotine in various biological samples, making it possible to identify nicotine poisoning as a cause of death. The presence of nicotine in non-smokers or unusually high levels in smokers can be a red flag in forensic investigations.

Historical Use: Historically, before the development of advanced forensic techniques, nicotine had been used more frequently in poisonings due to its easy extraction from tobacco leaves and the difficulty in detecting it as the cause of death.

Broader Implications of Nicotine Poisoning

Awareness of Toxicity: Cases like the 2014 murder highlight the toxic potential of substances commonly perceived as harmful only due to their addictive properties. It underscores the fact that many commonly used substances can be weaponized.

Regulatory Aspects: The incident also brings attention to the regulation of nicotine, especially in its pure form, which is highly concentrated and can be lethal.

Public Perception: While nicotine is most commonly associated with smoking-related health issues, cases of nicotine poisoning serve as a reminder of its inherent toxicity and potential for misuse.

Botulinum Toxin: From Cosmetic to Chemical Weapon

Botulinum Toxin in Context

Potent Neurotoxin: Botulinum toxin, produced by the bacterium Clostridium botulinum, is one of the most potent neurotoxins known to science. It causes botulism, a severe form of food poisoning, primarily when improperly canned or preserved foods are consumed.

Cosmetic Applications: In modern times, botulinum toxin has gained immense popularity for its cosmetic use, particularly in the form of Botox injections. These are used to reduce facial wrinkles by temporarily paralyzing muscles.

Concerns as a Bioweapon

Potential for Misuse: Given its potency, there has been longstanding concern about the potential misuse of botulinum toxin as a bioweapon. It could be dispersed as an aerosol or introduced into food or water supplies, posing a significant risk to public health.

Historical Research in Warfare: During World War II and the Cold War, several countries researched the potential of botulinum toxin as a biological warfare agent. The toxin's ability to cause widespread illness and death at extremely low concentrations made it an area of interest for bioweapons programs.

Regulation and Control: Due to these concerns, botulinum toxin is classified as a Category A bioterrorism agent by the Centers for Disease Control and Prevention (CDC) in the United States. This classification is reserved for pathogens that pose the highest risk to national security and public health.

Fewer Known Cases in Individual Murders

Challenges in Using as a Murder Weapon: Despite its potency, there are fewer documented cases of botulinum toxin being used in individual murders. This lower incidence is likely due to the difficulty in obtaining and handling the toxin, as well as its notoriety and the immediate suspicion it would arouse in cases of sudden and severe illness.

Detection and Forensic Investigation: Advances in forensic toxicology have made the detection of botulinum toxin in biological specimens more feasible, which could serve as a deterrent for its use in covert poisonings.

Broader Implications

Public Health and Safety: The potential misuse of botulinum toxin highlights the importance of stringent safety and regulatory measures in handling and distributing this substance, especially in its concentrated form.

Biomedical Research: The study of botulinum toxin has also contributed to the field of neuroscience, helping scientists understand more about nerve-muscle interactions and leading to the development of treatments for certain muscular disorders.

Emergency Preparedness: The threat posed by botulinum toxin underscores the need for preparedness in public health systems to respond to potential bioterrorism incidents.

16. The Race Against Time: Fighting Poisons with Science

Critical Timing in Administering Antidotes

Window of Opportunity: The period immediately following exposure to a poison is often crucial. The body's response to a toxin can be swift and severe, so the timely administration of an antidote can mean the difference between life and death.

Rapid Diagnosis and Response: Accurate and prompt diagnosis of the type of poisoning is essential for effective treatment. Emergency responders and healthcare professionals are trained to quickly identify poisoning symptoms and administer the appropriate antidote.

Challenges in Delayed Cases: In cases where there is a delay in treatment, the effectiveness of antidotes can be significantly reduced, and the risk of long-term damage or fatality increases.

Mechanisms of Action of Antidotes

Direct Neutralization: Some antidotes work by directly neutralizing the toxic effects of a poison. For instance, chelating agents like dimercaprol bind to heavy metals in the bloodstream, rendering them harmless.

Preventing Absorption: Activated charcoal is a common antidote that prevents the absorption of many poisons from the digestive system. It acts by binding to the toxin, thereby reducing its uptake into the bloodstream.

Physiological Antagonism: Certain antidotes act by counteracting the physiological effects of a toxin. For example, atropine, used in organophosphate poisoning, blocks the action of acetylcholine, a neurotransmitter that is overstimulated by organophosphates.

Enhancing Toxin Elimination: Some antidotes accelerate the elimination of toxins from the body. Sodium thiosulfate, used in cyanide poisoning, helps convert cyanide into a less toxic substance that can be more easily excreted.

Examples in Emergency Medicine

Naloxone for Opioid Overdoses: Naloxone is a life-saving antidote in cases of opioid overdose. It quickly reverses the effects of opioid drugs, restoring normal respiration in individuals whose breathing has slowed or stopped.

Atropine for Organophosphate Poisoning: Organophosphates, found in certain pesticides and nerve agents, can be lethal. Atropine, by inhibiting acetylcholine, helps alleviate symptoms like muscle weakness, convulsions, and respiratory distress.

Acetylcysteine for Acetaminophen Overdose: Acetaminophen (paracetamol) overdose is a common cause of liver failure. Acetylcysteine works by replenishing glutathione, a substance needed to detoxify the harmful metabolite of acetaminophen.

Famous Antidotes and Their Histories:

Mithridatism: Building Immunity Against Poisons

Historical Background: Named after Mithridates VI, the King of Pontus in the 1st century BC, mithridatism refers to the practice of building immunity to a poison by gradually self-administering non-lethal amounts. Mithridates, known for his fear of being poisoned, allegedly used this method to protect himself.

Legacy and Mythology: The story of Mithridates has taken on a legendary status over time, symbolizing the human quest for invulnerability against threats. Mithridatism inspired early toxicologists and physicians to explore the concept of immunity and tolerance to toxins.

Modern Perspective: In modern times, the concept of mithridatism is seen as dangerous and largely unfeasible due to the unpredictable nature of the body's response to different toxins.

Atropine and Organophosphates: A Life-Saving Antagonist

Source and Discovery: Atropine is an alkaloid derived from the deadly nightshade plant, Atropa belladonna. Its medicinal properties have been known since ancient times, but its use as an antidote to organophosphate poisoning is a 20th-century development.

Mechanism of Action: Organophosphates inhibit the enzyme acetylcholinesterase, leading to an accumulation of the neurotransmitter acetylcholine. Atropine works by blocking acetylcholine receptors, countering the effects of organophosphate poisoning.

Widespread Use: Atropine's effectiveness has made it a standard treatment in cases of pesticide and nerve agent poisoning. It is often carried in emergency kits by military personnel and first responders in areas where exposure to nerve agents is a risk.

Vitamin K and Warfarin: Antidote to an Anticoagulant

Warfarin's Dual Roles: Initially developed as a rat poison, warfarin later became an important anticoagulant medication used to prevent blood clots. Its discovery was prompted by investigations into a mysterious bleeding disease affecting cattle, which was eventually traced to a compound in spoiled sweet clover.

Vitamin K as an Antidote: Vitamin K acts as an antidote to warfarin overdose. Warfarin works by inhibiting vitamin K-dependent clotting factors. In cases of excessive anticoagulation, vitamin K is administered to restore the body's ability to form blood clots.

Medical Relevance: The relationship between warfarin and vitamin K is a classic example in medicine and pharmacology, illustrating the delicate balance required in anticoagulant therapy and the importance of antidotes in managing medication overdoses.

The histories of these antidotes not only reflect the evolution of medical science and our understanding of toxicology but also underscore the ongoing challenge of balancing the beneficial uses of substances with their potential risks. From ancient practices to modern medical treatments, the development of antidotes continues to be a crucial aspect of healthcare and emergency medicine.

The Challenges and Future of Antidote Research

Research Limitations in Antidote Development

Ethical Considerations: Testing new antidotes poses significant ethical challenges, especially when it comes to human trials. Ethical guidelines strictly regulate the administration of potentially harmful substances to humans, even in a controlled research setting.

Complexity and Cost: Developing an antidote is often a complex process involving extensive research, including the study of the toxin's mechanism of action, the antidote's interaction with human physiology, and potential side effects. This research can be incredibly time-consuming and expensive, requiring significant investment and resources.

Regulatory Hurdles: Navigating the regulatory landscape for approval of new antidotes can be challenging. Strict regulations and the need for comprehensive clinical trials to demonstrate efficacy and safety can delay the availability of lifesaving antidotes.

Broad-Spectrum Antidotes

Universal Antidote Concept: The idea of a universal or broad-spectrum antidote is an ongoing area of research. Such an antidote would be capable of neutralizing or mitigating the effects of a wide range of toxins.

Applications in Chemical Warfare and Bioterrorism: The development of broad-spectrum antidotes is particularly relevant in the context of chemical warfare and bioterrorism, where the nature of the toxin used may not be immediately known.

Challenges: The diversity of chemical structures and mechanisms of action among different toxins makes creating a truly broad-spectrum antidote extremely challenging.

Nanotechnology and Antidotes

Targeted Delivery Systems: Nanotechnology offers promising avenues for antidote development, particularly in creating targeted delivery systems that can transport antidotes directly to the affected organ or site of toxin action.

Enhanced Efficacy and Reduced Side Effects: Nanoparticles can potentially increase the efficacy of antidotes while minimizing side effects by ensuring that the antidote acts only where it is needed.

Innovative Approaches: Research is exploring the use of nanoparticles to sequester toxins or to act as carriers for enzymes or other molecules that can neutralize toxins.

Genetic and Molecular Approaches

Personalized Medicine in Toxicology: Genetic and molecular techniques are paving the way for more personalized approaches to antidote therapy. Understanding an individual's genetic response to certain toxins could lead to more effective and personalized treatments.

Mechanistic Insights: Advances in molecular biology are providing deeper insights into how toxins interact with human cells and organs at the molecular level, opening up possibilities for new antidote mechanisms.

Potential for Genetic Therapies: There is potential for developing genetic therapies that could either enhance the body's natural detoxification processes or directly counteract the effects of specific toxins.

The future of antidote research holds significant promise, driven by advances in technology and a deeper understanding of toxicology and human biology. While challenges remain, particularly in terms of ethical considerations and the complexity of antidote development, the ongoing research is crucial for addressing both existing and emerging threats from toxins and poisons.

17. Poison in Pop Culture

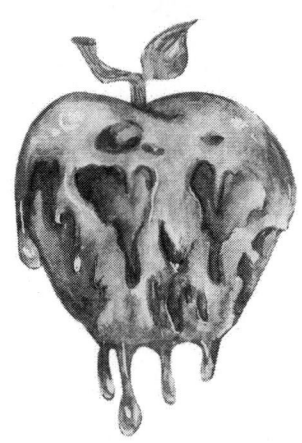

Introduction to Poison in Popular Culture

The allure of poison has captivated the imagination of artists, writers, and filmmakers for centuries. In popular culture, poison is often depicted as a tool of intrigue, mystery, and drama. Its silent, hidden nature makes it a perfect device for plot twists in stories, symbolizing both the ingenuity and malevolence of characters. This chapter explores how poison has been portrayed in literature, movies, and TV shows, drawing parallels between famous fictional poisonings and their real-world counterparts.

Portrayal of Poison in Literature:

    Classic Literature: From Shakespeare's tragic plays, where characters like King Claudius in

"Hamlet" and Lady Macbeth in "Macbeth" use poison as a means to their nefarious ends, to Agatha Christie's murder mysteries like "A Pocket Full of Rye" where poison becomes a central plot device, literature is replete with toxic substances.

Symbolism and Themes: Poison in literature often symbolizes betrayal, secrecy, and the darker aspects of human nature. It's used to navigate themes of power, revenge, and justice. For instance, in Alexandre Dumas' "The Count of Monte Cristo," poison is a tool for vengeance and retribution.

Poison in Movies and TV Shows:

Dramatic Storytelling: In movies and TV, poison is used for its dramatic effect. Films like "Arsenic and Old Lace" and "The Princess Bride" use poison in central plotlines, combining dark humor with suspense.

Visual Representation: The depiction of poison in visual media often involves dramatic scenes of characters suffering or intricate plots revolving around the administration of the poison. The TV series "Breaking Bad," for instance, effectively uses the poison ricin to build tension and advance the plot.

Character Development: In many films and TV series, the choice of poison and the method of its administration are used to develop characters. A sophisticated villain might use a rare, untraceable poison, while a more brutish antagonist might opt for a more violent method of poisoning.

Famous Fictional Poisonings and Real-World Counterparts:

Iocane Powder in "The Princess Bride": This fictional poison, famed for being odorless, tasteless, and dissolving instantly in liquid, is used in a memorable battle of wits. Real-life counterparts might include poisons like arsenic or ricin, known for their potency and difficulty to detect.

Joffrey's Death in "Game of Thrones": The poisoning of King Joffrey with "The Strangler" – a fictional poison that causes asphyxiation – mirrors real toxins that disrupt the body's physiological functions, such as cyanide.

Gustave H's Death in "Grand Budapest Hotel": The use of poison in Wes Anderson's film aligns with historical uses of poison, where it was often employed discreetly to eliminate rivals or secure power.

Conclusion: The Enduring Fascination with Poison

The representation of poison in popular culture reflects a deep human fascination with the power of substances that can alter or end life surreptitiously. From the works of Shakespeare to modern TV thrillers, poison remains a compelling element, embodying the complexities of human emotions and motivations. Its portrayal in pop culture not only entertains but also educates, offering insights into both the creative human psyche and the darker corners of human actions. This chapter underscores how the narrative of poison continues to evolve, mirroring changes in societal norms, scientific understanding, and artistic expression.

18. The Modern Age of Poisoning

Introduction to Contemporary Trends in Poisoning

In the modern age, the landscape of poisoning has undergone significant changes. The evolution from natural poisons derived from plants and animals to sophisticated synthetic toxins has dramatically altered the scope and nature of poisoning. This chapter explores this shift, the emergence of chemical warfare, and notable contemporary poisoning incidents, examining their broader societal implications.

The Shift from Natural to Synthetic Poisons

Historical Context: Traditionally, poisons were derived from natural sources like plants (belladonna, hemlock), animals (snake venom), and minerals (arsenic, mercury). These substances were often used for personal vendettas, political assassinations, and even medical treatments.

Synthetic Revolution: The 20th century saw a revolution in chemistry that led to the synthesis of new, potent toxins. Advances in organic chemistry enabled the creation of compounds like sarin, VX nerve agent, and various pharmaceuticals that could be used as poisons.

Enhanced Potency and Precision: Synthetic poisons offer a level of potency and specificity that natural toxins often lack. They can be engineered to target specific biological systems and have predictable effects, making them more controllable and, in some ways, more dangerous.

The Rise of Chemical Warfare and Its Implications

Development and Use: The use of chemical weapons in warfare, notably during World War I and II, marked a dark chapter in the history of conflict. Agents like mustard gas, phosgene, and nerve agents were employed, causing horrific injuries and deaths.

International Treaties and Bans: The devastating impact of chemical weapons led to international treaties banning their use, such as the Geneva Protocol and the Chemical Weapons Convention. However, compliance and enforcement remain challenges.

Ethical and Moral Dilemmas: The development and potential use of chemical weapons pose profound ethical and moral dilemmas. They represent the dark side of scientific advancement, where knowledge that could be used for good is turned into instruments of harm.

Contemporary Poisoning Incidents and Their Societal Impact

Notable Cases: In recent decades, high-profile poisoning cases have grabbed headlines, such as the use of polonium-210 in the assassination of Alexander Litvinenko, the nerve agent attack on Sergei and Yulia Skripal in Salisbury, and the murder of Kim Jong-nam using VX nerve agent.

Terrorism and Criminal Acts: The modern era has seen the use of poisons in acts of terrorism and criminal activities. The accessibility of certain synthetic toxins and the knowledge to produce them have raised concerns about their use by non-state actors and individuals.

Public Awareness and Anxiety: These incidents have heightened public awareness and anxiety regarding the use of poisons. They underscore the need for vigilance, improved detection methods, and emergency preparedness to respond to poisoning cases.

Forensic Advances: Modern forensic science has evolved to detect and analyze poisons with greater accuracy and speed. This has been crucial in solving crimes and implementing safety measures.

Navigating the Modern Landscape of Poisoning

The modern age of poisoning reflects a complex interplay between scientific progress, ethical considerations, and societal impacts. While the development of synthetic poisons has expanded the boundaries of chemistry and medicine, it has also introduced new risks and challenges. The transition from natural to synthetic toxins, the specter of chemical warfare, and notable poisoning incidents shape our understanding of the role of poisons in the contemporary world. This chapter highlights the importance of continued vigilance, ethical responsibility, and scientific inquiry in the realm of toxicology.

19. Conclusion: The Enduring Enigma of Poisons

Reflection on the Dual Nature of Poisons

A Double-Edged Sword: The history of poisons is a testament to their dual nature. On one hand, they have been used as tools for murder, political assassinations, and warfare. On the other, they have served as the basis for life-saving medications and medical treatments. This duality is at the heart of the enigma surrounding poisons.

From Harm to Healing: Many substances that were historically used as poisons have found their place in modern medicine. For instance, botulinum toxin, once a feared poison, is now used in therapeutic treatments for various muscular disorders. Similarly, compounds like digitalis, derived from the poisonous foxglove plant, are used to treat heart conditions.

Ethical and Moral Considerations: The history of poisons brings to light the ethical and moral questions inherent in the use of these substances. It challenges us to consider the fine line between harm and healing and the responsibilities that come with the knowledge of toxicology.

The Future: The Evolving Science and Study of Poisons

Advancements in Toxicology: The field of toxicology is continually evolving, with new discoveries and technologies enhancing our understanding of how poisons interact with biological systems. Advanced analytical techniques and computer modeling are paving the way for more precise and comprehensive studies of toxic substances.

Emerging Challenges: In the modern world, we face new challenges in the realm of poisons. The development of synthetic chemicals and environmental pollutants, the threat of bioterrorism, and the potential misuse of toxic substances in a globalized world require ongoing vigilance and adaptation in the field of toxicology.

Education and Awareness: Public education and awareness about poisons and their effects are crucial in preventing accidental poisonings and intentional misuse. Educating individuals about the safe handling of potentially toxic substances and the importance of poison control measures is an integral part of public health.

Interdisciplinary Approaches: The study of poisons today is an interdisciplinary endeavor, involving chemistry, biology, medicine, environmental science, and even ethics and law. This collaborative approach is essential in addressing the complex issues surrounding poisons in our society.

Poisons, with their capacity to harm and to heal, continue to fascinate and challenge humanity. Their study is not just about understanding the substances themselves but also about exploring the broader implications for health, society, and ethics. As we look to the future, the field of toxicology stands at the forefront of scientific advancement, balancing the potential risks and benefits of these powerful substances. The enduring enigma of poisons is a reminder of the ever-present need for responsible science, informed policy, and a deep respect for both the power and the peril they represent.

20. Appendix

Glossary of Terms

- **Acetylcholinesterase**: An enzyme that breaks down acetylcholine, a neurotransmitter. Inhibited by certain poisons like organophosphates.

- **Chelation Therapy**: A treatment used to remove heavy metals from the bloodstream, often used in cases of lead or mercury poisoning.

- **Cyanogenic Glycosides**: Naturally occurring compounds found in certain plants that can release cyanide when metabolized.

- **Hemlock**: A poisonous plant, famous for its use in the execution of Socrates.

- **LD50**: Lethal Dose 50, a standard measure of a substance's toxicity, indicating the dose required to kill 50% of a test population.

- **Mithridatism**: The practice of building immunity to a poison by gradually self-administering non-lethal amounts.

- **Neurotoxin**: A toxin that acts specifically on nerve cells (neurons), usually by disrupting their function.

- **Ricin**: A highly toxic protein derived from the castor bean plant.

- **Toxicology**: The study of the adverse effects of chemicals on living organisms.

- **Xenobiotic**: A chemical substance that is foreign to the biological system.

Timeline of Key Poisoning Incidents

- **399 BC**: Socrates executed by hemlock poisoning.
- **AD 54**: Roman Emperor Claudius allegedly poisoned with mushrooms.
- **1834**: Birth of Mathieu Orfila, considered the father of modern toxicology.
- **1850s**: Arsenic wallpapers cause widespread health issues.
- **1978**: Georgi Markov assassinated with a ricin-laced pellet.
- **1982**: Chicago Tylenol murders, leading to safety seals on consumer products.
- **1995**: Tokyo subway sarin attack.
- **2006**: Alexander Litvinenko poisoned with polonium-210.
- **2017**: Assassination of Kim Jong-nam using VX nerve agent.

Recommended Reading and Resources

1. **"The Poisoner's Handbook" by Deborah Blum**: A gripping chronicle of the birth of forensic toxicology in Jazz Age New York.
2. **"Molecules of Murder" by John Emsley**: Explores some of the most notorious poisoning cases and the poisons involved.
3. **"The Secret Poisoner: A Century of Murder" by Linda Stratmann**: A detailed look at the history of poison and murder in the Victorian era.
4. **"Poisons: From Hemlock to Botox" by Peter Macinnis**: Offers an engaging overview of poisons throughout history.
5. **"The Elements of Murder: A History of Poison" by John Emsley**: An in-depth look at the five most deadly chemicals in history.

Online Resources

- **The International Programme on Chemical Safety (IPCS)**: Provides essential health and safety information on chemicals.

- **The American Association of Poison Control Centers (AAPCC)**: Offers resources and information on poison prevention and control.

These resources provide a comprehensive understanding of the role of poisons in history, medicine, and criminal investigations, offering both historical context and scientific insight.

Printed in Great Britain
by Amazon

67abdd9a-c638-42d5-8c98-2c418ab6da6aR01

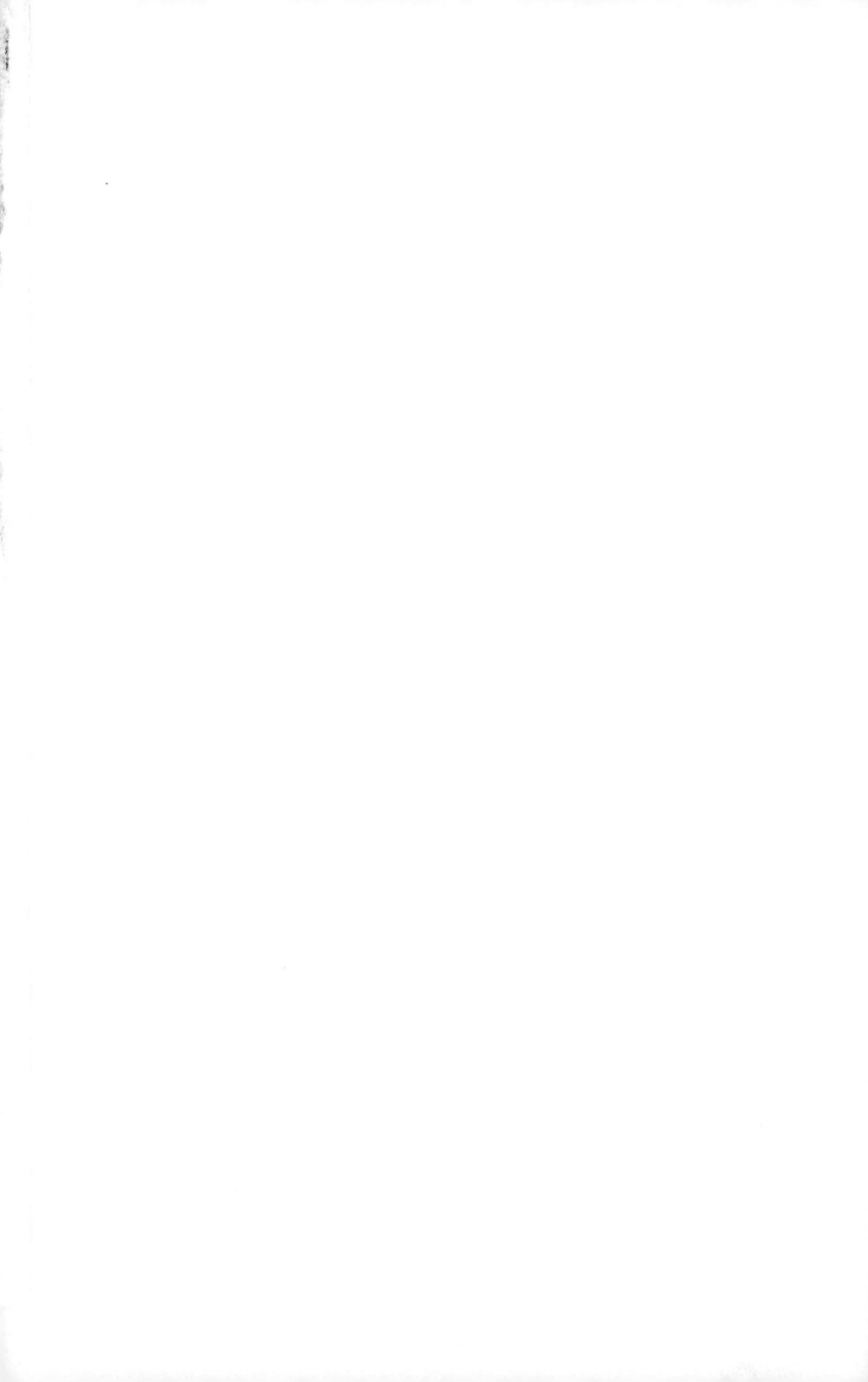